The Happiness Upgrade
One Small Step Up to a Happier Life

☙ 52-Week Journal Included ❧

Gabrielle Lichterman

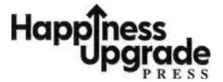

Jun 27, 2022

To Melanie & Brian,
I hope this book leads to many Happiness Upgrades in your lives.
xx, Gabrielle

Happiness
Upgrade
PRESS

The Happiness Upgrade
One Small Step Up to a Happier Life

Gabrielle Lichterman

Published by Happiness Upgrade Press, LLC
St. Petersburg, Florida, USA

ISBN: 978-1-7362353-2-4

The Happiness Upgrade is intended as a reference volume only, not as a medical manual. In light of the complex, individual, and specific nature of health problems, this book is not intended to replace professional medical advice. The ideas, procedures, and suggestions in this book are intended to supplement, not replace, the advice of a trained medical professional. Consult with your physician before adopting the suggestions in this book, as well as about any condition that may require diagnosis or medical attention. The author and publisher disclaim any liability arising directly or indirectly from the use of this book.
—Adapted from a *Declaration of Principles* jointly adopted by a Committee of the American Bar Association and a Committee of Publishers and Associations.

More Books by This Author

You might enjoy these other health and self-help books by Gabrielle Lichterman…

28 Days: What Your Cycle Reveals About Your Moods, Health and Potential
This groundbreaking book launched the popular movement to live in sync with the ups and downs of hormones in your menstrual cycle.

Hormonology Menstrual Cycle Tracker Journal
Tracking every facet of your menstrual cycle (from flow and basal temperature to mood and changes in health conditions) has never been easier—or more private—than with this comprehensive, customizable paperback menstrual cycle tracking journal.

Hormonology Day-by-Day Menstrual Cycle Guided Journal
In this guided daily journal, you'll learn how to pinpoint the hormonal strengths and challenges specific to your menstrual cycle. Plus, you get inspirational messages that help you harness the positive power of your hormones.

DIY Résumé and Cover Letter Kit: Everything You Need to Create Your Own Professional-Quality Résumé and Cover Letter
You don't need to spend a bundle to get a résumé and cover letter that look like they were written by a pro. This simple step-by-step guide shows you how to easily create them yourself.

To learn more about these books and forthcoming books, visit GabrielleLichterman.com.

Table of Contents

Preface:
Small Changes=Big Results

The Happiness Upgrade doesn't promise euphoric joy in an instant. Or a day. Or even a week. It won't plaster a smile on your face 24/7 or insist you smile when you're not feeling it. It can't instantly fix stressful jobs, mend unhappy relationships or cure illnesses. It won't magically make sadness disappear or ask you to mask negative emotions.

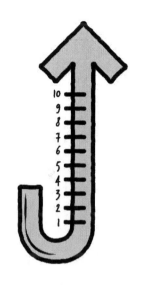

What this book offers is much more realistic, but extraordinarily useful: It introduces you to the **Happiness Upgrade** method. With it, you'll learn how to nudge up your mood just *one small step* on an imaginary happiness scale of **1** to **10**, where **1** is the lowest mood and **10** is the highest. For example, you'll learn how to go from a **1** to a **2**. A **4** to a **5**. An **8** to a **9**. And so on.

This one small step up is a more powerful tool than it may at first seem. That's because it can…

- Pause a negative mood, preventing a downward spiral into a worse mood
- Spur an upward spiral into a better mood
- Make challenging situations, people or moments easier to handle, reducing stress
- Inspire you to discover quick, easy methods that help you cope with life's challenges, boosting resilience
- Enhance the pleasure you get from positive experiences, making them even more joy-inducing

Best of all, the **Happiness Upgrade** method is easy to use every day. That's because it…

- Works in seconds and can be implemented virtually anywhere, anytime
- Is small enough to be easy to do, yet powerful enough to impact your mood
- Can lead you to rising one more step up the happiness scale, then another, so you continue your upward spiral, boosting your mood even higher

If you're ready to discover the ease and power of giving yourself a **Happiness Upgrade**, read on. Here's what you'll get in this book:

- You'll learn the simple **Happiness Upgrade** method and how to apply it
- You'll be given a 52-week journal to track how you've used the **Happiness Upgrade** method in your life so you can pinpoint the best **Happiness Upgrades** that work specifically for you
- You'll get inspiration from 52 study-backed **Happiness Upgrade** suggestions that can help move your mood one step up on the happiness scale

Introduction:
How I Developed the
Happiness Upgrade Method

[Trigger warning: Text includes references to depression and suicidal ideation.]

From my adolescence to my early 20s, I struggled with severe depression. This was during the 1980s and early 1990s, a time when this kind of health condition came with more challenges than it does today: Finding a qualified therapist, doctor or medication to successfully treat depression was woefully difficult; the Internet was in its contentless, dial-up infancy offering zero help; and, depression carried more stigma, often kept a deep, dark secret from family and friends.

So, looking back it was no surprise that my numerous attempts at treatment didn't work. Antidepressants were relatively new and my doctor wasn't well-versed in how to use them. The kind of talk therapy that therapists tried left me feeling worse after every session. And, I didn't have anyone close in my life that I felt comfortable confiding in to ask for help.

Then, at the age of 23, I faced a new challenge that made my already severe depression grow in intensity, forcing me to find a solution no matter what.

Life takes a downward turn

While living in Greenwich Village in Manhattan, I was in two accidents resulting in concussions within the space of just a few months: The first head trauma was when I lost my footing and fell down a slippery flight of stairs, hitting the back of my skull on every step on the way down. The second concussion occurred when I was riding in the back of a taxi. The driver rear-ended another taxi at full speed, propelling my forehead into the Plexiglass divider.

1

Fueled by two successive brain injuries, my depression darkened to a point I never imagined it could go. Every day became more hopeless than the last. Then one day I woke up, loaded a bullet into the chamber of an old rifle I'd kept in a closet and knew if I didn't get help right away, this would be the last morning I'd see.

Somehow, I summoned the will to head to the nearest emergency room and let them know I was in a depressed, suicidal state. They bundled me into an ambulance and deposited me at a well-known psychiatric hospital a couple of miles from my apartment.

I voluntarily checked myself in. The desk nurse took away all my belongings and shoelaces. Then I was led to a small, dingy room that was bare except for two empty twin beds. It reeked of disinfectant and human waste. There were two windows that were too high to see out of and were covered in a tight crisscross of bars, barely allowing any sunlight to shine through. I was told a doctor would be with me shortly.

Eight hours later, I was still sitting on the same twin bed in the same stuffy, smelly room alone. No one had checked on me. I hadn't even been offered food or water. The sensation of being discarded and forgotten in my weakest moment felt like a crushing kick in the gut. Hungry, thirsty, bored and hopeless, I stood up and checked myself out of the hospital.

Because I was there voluntarily, no one blocked me from leaving. I was surprised to discover that it was as easy to depart as checking out of a hotel. However, I was told I would have to return the next day for my wallet, keys and shoelaces since the nurse with access to patient belongings had left hours earlier.

By the time I got out of the hospital, it was nighttime. Without my wallet, I couldn't get on the subway or take a bus. So, I walked the two miles back to my apartment building in lace-less sneakers that flopped like circus clown shoes with each step. I knocked on my neighbor's door and asked for the spare key I once gave him so I could let myself in. Then, I was back in the same apartment where I'd been holding a loaded gun to my mouth that same morning. I picked up the rifle and put it back in the closet.

The plan

After gobbling whatever food I had in the kitchen and gulping down glass after glass of water to rehydrate, I sat quietly. My emotions revolved like a merry-go-round, spinning from humiliation to despair to anger to resentment. But, in between I couldn't help laughing at the absurdity of what I experienced that day.

Ultimately, I came to the conclusion that I'd officially run out of avenues to look for help. And worse, asking for assistance from others was having the *opposite* effect—it was making me feel more hopeless every time it failed. It became obvious to me that I had hit my "bottom" and if I wanted to climb out of this deep pit of depression (and I sincerely did), I would need to rely on myself.

So, over the next few hours, I made a plan: I committed to getting healthier. I'd start by eating more nutritious food. No more junk food and fast food for breakfast, lunch and dinner. I'd stick to a regular sleep schedule and clock seven to eight hours of sleep at night rather than stay up 'til dawn and erratically squeeze in a couple of hours of shuteye here and there. I'd adopt an exercise regimen and get in shape. And, I'd give up alcohol, which I knew was a depressant, but was also leaning on as a self-medicating crutch. I had a strong hunch that getting physically healthier would get me mentally healthier.

My plan was ambitious and called for many dramatic changes. When you're challenged with depression, finding the motivation to make just *one* positive change can be an excruciating feat. But, having exhausted every other path available to me, I knew this might be my last option. So, I mustered every ounce of energy I had left and gave it my all.

Slowly over a few months, my brain responded. My plan worked! For me, healthier did, indeed, mean happier. This motivated me to continue to stick to my healthy habits, which continued to help my depression lift. I felt like I was finally crawling out of the black hole that had enveloped me for so many years. It was the kind of relief I'd been hoping for.

Preventing a relapse

Even though my mood was getting significantly brighter, I'd soon learn that once you get depression under control, it doesn't necessarily mean it goes away permanently. Instead, it can be like some types of cancer: it goes into remission. I discovered mine could reappear due to stress, resuming unhealthy lifestyle habits or simply for no good reason at all.

Because of this, I realized I needed to add tips to my depression-fighting plan to help me avoid a relapse. I developed some useful tactics:

- Strike a work/life balance to lower stress
- Notice when I'm developing an unhealthy habit, such as not sleeping seven to eight hours nightly, then correct it
- Change my exercise routine if it became too monotonous to stick to

A piece of the puzzle was missing

While my plan felt fairly comprehensive, I realized there was still one crucial element missing: I needed a way to halt sadness, rumination, anxiety, stress, anger, pessimism or embarrassment the moment it crept in. This way, I could slam the brakes on a negative spiral down that could lead me to another bout of depression.

Optimally, the technique would also boost my mood at least a little so I could turn the ship around and start spiraling up.

On top of that, the technique needed to be something simple that I could use anywhere, anytime. I didn't want to have to wait to get home or hold off until a stressful situation was over to use it. And, it had to be something I could do as easily in a crowded room as I could alone.

My goal wasn't to become deliriously happy, which is unrealistic. And, I didn't want to adopt a fake-it-'til-you-make-it form of "toxic positivity" where you pretend to be upbeat when you aren't. I needed to genuinely feel just a little better. And to genuinely feel just a little better *right now*.

Of course, I knew this was a lot to ask, but that didn't deter me from working hard to find the perfect solution. I experimented with a whole host of tactics that didn't end up panning out. For example, I tried perking myself up with self-massage (but realized you can't do that while carrying two armfuls of groceries down a busy Manhattan street), inhaling a pleasant aroma (but kept forgetting to put a favorite essential oil in my purse for times I needed it) and treating myself to a cup of herbal tea (but could only do that when I was home with my kettle or happened to be near a deli).

The experiments dragged on for months. No single tactic fit all my criteria. Then one day, the perfect solution finally hit me.

The Happiness Upgrade method is invented

I didn't need to find one specific coping tactic to use over and over in every situation. I needed to find one *type* of coping tactic. Then, I could use different tactics that fit the moment to make any situation just a little better. For example, if I was on a subway that was stuck in a tunnel, that's when I could give myself a hand or neck massage to help ease the frustration. If I was feeling exhausted while walking down a city street with my arms full of groceries, that's when I could put down my shopping bags for a moment in front of a flower stand, then take a whiff of a fragrant rose, which I knew would lift my spirits. If I was stressed about a deadline while working at home, that's when I could brew myself a hot cup of herbal tea.

The collective scope of all the ways I could eke out a small mood boost anywhere, anytime was the exact coping method I needed. Since my goal was to get an upgrade in good feelings, I named my newfound method the **Happiness Upgrade**.

And, it worked! Aiming to get just a smidgen happier made stressful moments more bearable. Anxious times a tad calmer. Embarrassing slip-ups easier to put behind me. And sad spells just a little lighter. This not only prevented a downward emotional spiral, it propelled me up in a more positive direction.

But, then I discovered this **Happiness Upgrade** had other benefits.

Giving myself a **Happiness Upgrade** helped make ordinary moments—not sad or stressed, just meh—more pleasant. It was easier to notice a comforting breeze on a sunny day or smile from a passing stranger. It spurred me to treat myself to a cup of cocoa or put a flower in a bud vase on my desk. It reminded me to add more moments of positivity to my day, which made my overall day better.

It also inspired me to make extraordinary moments even more enjoyable. For instance, when watching beautiful sunsets from my apartment building roof, I'd take a lawn chair so I could sit down and relax as I watched the sun dip below the city's skyline.

The Happiness Upgrade 25 years later

Twenty-five years ago, transforming my own mental health inspired me to devote my then fledgling writing career to health journalism. I wanted to show others how they could also improve their well-being by becoming an active member of their own healthcare team. Sure, doctors, nurses, therapists and other medical professionals are vitally important. And, thankfully, the healthcare field has made significant advancements with treatments for depression and other mental health conditions over the years. But, as I've experienced personally, patients also have the power to improve their own health.

Helping others find out how to become a valuable member of their own healthcare team has been one my key driving forces as a professional journalist. And, it seems that folks appreciate the guidance: I've written thousands of health articles for major publications around the globe. I'm also an award-winning author who pioneered a form of health management followed by millions, called **Hormonology**, that helps women harness the power of the hormones in their menstrual cycle.

Now I'm introducing a technique that I've been using personally for more than 25 years to help you manage your moods. It's designed specifically to help you pause and reverse "toxic" negativity—the kind of anger, sadness and other emotion that can worsen mental health issues or raise your risk of developing them.

It's important to note that some temporary negative moods are helpful, for example, anger at a fellow employee who's stealing your work and presenting it as their own can motivate you to stand up for yourself. Grief helps you process a loss. And, regret helps you learn from mistakes.

The primary goal of the **Happiness Upgrade** method is to help you manage *unhealthy* negative moods that can lead to a downward spiral. For example, it can ease anger that's out of proportion for a situation, help you climb out of ongoing sadness and pause the pain of embarrassment.

The **Happiness Upgrade** isn't a cure for depression, anxiety or other mental health conditions. And, what worked for my depression may not necessarily work for yours. However, this easy technique can be one of the tools you try as a complement to your current treatment or to help you manage your moods, in general.

Read on in this book to…

- Find out what the **Happiness Upgrade** method is
- Discover why it works so well to boost mood
- Learn how to easily incorporate it into your own life
- Get study-backed **Happiness Upgrade** suggestions to start using the method right away
- Log your own personal **Happiness Upgrades**

I'm not an academic proposing a new theory of overnight personal transformation. I'm a longtime health journalist who has been challenged by depression and developed a simple technique to boost mood in the moment. It's worked for me and folks I know. Now I'm sharing it with you so it can possibly help you, too.

Please note: If you're feeling suicidal or have thoughts of self-harm, please contact your doctor or therapist, talk with a loved one or call a suicide hotline. My experience was not typical. Help is available.

Chapter 1:
Spiraling Down or Spiraling Up?

As humans, we're constantly in motion. We move forward in line and move backward to avoid getting splashed by someone's hot cup of coffee. We go up escalators, down elevators and stride through moving walkways in the airport. We cross streets, climb hills and run in circles. We step into cars, hop into planes, traverse in trains and ride our bikes, roller skates, scooters and skateboards with abandon. When we sleep, we're still tossing and turning. There's just no stopping us. Even when we're sitting down, the stuff inside us—blood, hormones, immune cells, oxygen, waste—is constantly on the move.

In a similar way, your mood is also continually moving, heading either up or down. And, it's often due to situations you don't expect or can't control. For instance...

> *While in a grocery store, out of nowhere, someone accidentally runs over your foot with their shopping cart—and boom!—your mood suddenly goes down.*

> *While in a grocery store, you unexpectedly discover they now stock your favorite cookies that you haven't been able to find in years—and boom!—your mood suddenly goes up.*

When you experience a change in mood—up or down—due to some kind of experience or situation, it doesn't just stop there. Your mood tends to continue to move in that same direction. So, if your mood goes down, it typically continues to go down. If your mood goes up, it typically continues to move up. For example...

> *After your mood goes down because your foot was rolled over by a shopping cart, you become more easily frustrated by the long line at the grocery check-out, which makes you even more annoyed.*

After your mood goes up because you discovered your favorite cookies are now being stocked at the grocery store, you rave about your sweet discovery to the cashier at the check-out and enjoy the friendly conversation you have with her, then leave the store with an even bigger smile.

The downward mood spiral

It's not your fault that once your mood starts to fall, it continues to drop. It's not due to lack of willpower. You don't have a defect. You didn't do anything wrong. Truth is, once your mood starts to go south, it tends to continue heading further down on its own.

Why? Honestly, and perhaps frustratingly, is that it's just the way humans are wired. Once you experience a situation that causes aggravation, anger, embarrassment, irritability, regret, sadness or another negative emotion, it triggers changes in the body that make this negative emotional state last long after the situation is over. For example, your body pumps out certain chemicals that impact mood, such as anger-fueling adrenaline. And, areas of the brain that manage emotion behave differently, prolonging the negative feelings.

Along with this, when your mood drops, it can cause changes throughout the rest of your body that keep an unwanted emotion going. For instance, your muscles tend to tense up when you're angry and you tend slouch when you're sad. These postures send signals to the brain, telling it that you're in an angry or sad mood, which then prompts your body to churn out more chemicals to match that negative feeling, making it linger.[1]

Making matters worse, new negative experiences can trigger vivid memories of past unpleasant experiences. Researchers suspect it's because we evolved to recall harmful situations as a way to avoid them in the future.[2]

Now let's go back to the grocery store example to show how all of this plays out in a real-life scenario…

9

Your foot accidentally gets run over by a grocery cart because of a distracted shopper. Immediately, your adrenaline rises, which tenses up muscles. You determine it was an accident. The shopper may have even apologized. However, you also quickly realize that your foot hurts. It's not broken but, dang, it smarts! So, now you get a bigger spike in adrenaline, which intensifies your irritation, turning it into outright anger that you now have at the hapless shopper. You probably fume a bit. Sure, you accept their apology, but you might also mutter some choice words under your breath. Your muscles remain tensed as you continue your shopping, which might aggravate an old back injury, causing physical pain that makes you even more irritable. Perhaps, you start forcefully throwing groceries into your cart out of anger. Then, you toss in a glass bottle of salad dressing and it breaks, leaving a gloppy mess to clean up, infuriating you even more. Your mood continues to go down...

These negative feelings and actions are common. Unless you've been trained to keep your cool in any situation, for example, with mindfulness meditation or military preparation, most of us would have a similar reaction. It's just how humans are built. You get ticked off or sad or anxious or embarrassed, so now your body spurs changes that match that feeling, keeping you in that state.

As a result of these physical changes, if you don't do anything to pause your negative mood or turn it around, your mood typically continues to move in the same direction it's already headed—down. So, you get sadder, angrier or more embarrassed.

Of course, for most of us, this negative mood does eventually wear off. It may take a half-hour, an hour, a few hours or maybe even a whole day. However, for some, these bouts of negativity don't go away or go away completely, which can lead to a downward spiral of depression, anxiety, burnout or other serious mental health issues that lasts for days, weeks or months.

The upward mood spiral

Now say something good happens to you, such as discovering your grocery store has started stocking your favorite cookies that you haven't been able to find in years. You'll likely get surprised, excited and delighted. As a result, a grin probably spreads across your face. You might stop a passing shopper to rave about how great these cookies are to convince her to try them. And, you may buy extra boxes to pass out to friends and family.

These positive feelings are normal. It's just how humans are wired. You get happy, so your brain churns out more chemicals that match this happy feeling, such as endorphins and dopamine, keeping you upbeat.

On top of that, your own thoughts and actions while in this happy state can lead to more positive experiences that continue your upward mood spiral. For example, perhaps an elderly person sees your big smile, then smiles back you, which makes you feel even warmer inside. And, maybe the shopper you recommended the cookies to shares one of her favorite treats with you, so now you have another great item to put in your basket and look forward to enjoying. Then, maybe the friends and family who you gave your favorite cookies to reward you with hugs or they gift you with something from their pantry that they love.

Once your mood starts to go up, it launches an upward spiral that tends to continue.

The good news is that when an upward spiral continues on and on, it can chase off the blues, help ease depression, reduce anxiety, improve mental and physical energy, rev motivation, create a surge in optimism and give your life more meaning.

Move your mood in the right direction

You can see that it doesn't take a whole lot to send your mood spiraling up or down. One small event can have a dramatic, long-lasting impact on you.

But, that's a *good* thing! That's because it means you can harness this odd phenomenon to impact your own mood whenever you want. All it takes is doing small, easy actions to deliberately move your mood in an upward spiral.

And that's what the **Happiness Upgrade** method is all about.

You don't have to wait for positive events to randomly happen to you (like discovering your favorite cookies at the grocery store) to spur a better mood or pause a negative mood. You can do small acts anywhere, anytime that move your emotions in a positive direction, such as pouring yourself a cup of coffee, going outdoors for a one-minute break, sniffing a fragrant flower or turning on music you enjoy.

While these tiny acts may seem too insignificant to have any impact, they're enough of a nudge to get you moving in a happier direction. And, this is backed by research.

The science of small moves

For decades, researchers from around the globe have been investigating the power of doing small acts to achieve big mood-boosting results. In study after study, they've discovered that a small action you take can improve your mood in the present moment. Plus, it can help continue to push your mood in a positive direction so it keeps spiraling up. Following are a few examples of these studies...

- In 1998, social psychologist Barbara L. Fredrickson, Ph.D., introduced the "broaden-and-build" theory. In it, she proposed that experiencing positive emotions spurs an upward spiral of good feelings by building resources that make it easier to cope, leading to more positive experiences and more life satisfaction.[3] Fredrickson's subsequent studies confirmed her theory.[4]

- In 2009, reporting in the journal *Emotion*, a research team that included Fredrickson found that small positive "micro-moments" in your day (such as enjoying a cup of tea) are more important for happiness than more general life outcomes (such as your job or marital status) because they make you more resilient.[5]

- Reviews of studies that examined the effects of "positive activity interventions" (actions that improve mood and increase positive thinking) by research teams that included noted University of California happiness scientist Sonja Lyubomirsky, Ph.D., found that simple positive acts, such as counting your blessings, are such powerful mood enhancers, they can even help clinically depressed patients get an emotional lift.[6] That's because one small positive action spurs a domino effect: It provides a temporary mood boost that gives you the energy and motivation to pursue goals that increase positive emotions even more. For example, you might feel uplifted after watching an inspirational video, then channel that energy to sign up for a yoga class that you've been meaning to try where you then make new friends who lift good feelings even more.

- In a 2011 study that examined why shopping boosts mood, researchers from the University of Michigan found that it's primarily due to the small act of making choices, such as putting a sweater on a wish list.[7] That's because these micro-decisions give you a sense of control, which is a key component of feeling happier.

- In a 2015 study from Yale University and the University of Colorado at Boulder, investigators discovered that happy people notice more positive moments in their day, which fuels better well-being.[8] Soon after, scientists from Radboud University Nijmegen in the Netherlands published research showing that folks who aren't naturally inclined to notice positivity around them could learn to spot it, increasing their happiness, too.[9]

- Researchers reporting in the *Journal of Sport & Exercise Psychology* in 2021 found that athletes who had a pleasant experience (such as reading a motivational passage in a book) performed better immediately. What's more, this improvement in performance lasted into the following week.[10] That's because the initial mood boost made them open to using coping strategies that helped them deal with the pressures of competing, which lowered stress and kept their mood elevated.

Researchers have shown again and again that small acts have a positive effect on mood as you do them. Plus, they can spur an upward spiral of positive emotions, helping to increase good feelings as well as boost life satisfaction, well-being and resilience.

This means that even if you're in a difficult situation (such as having a stressful job or caring for of an ailing loved one), taking one small action to add a glimmer of positivity to your day can still help nudge your emotions in an upward direction.

And, if you're looking to add more sparks of happiness to an ordinary day, it's easier to achieve than you may have assumed.

Chapter 2:
The Happiness Upgrade Method

Decades of scientific research prove that taking a small, positive action has the power to nudge up your mood and keep it spiraling up. The **Happiness Upgrade** method adds an important tool to this science: It incorporates a simple **1** to **10** happiness scale that shows you *how* to take a small mood-boosting action whenever you need it.

It's like putting an imaginary ladder in your mind so you can focus on climbing up each rung one by one versus scaling up a wall with no tools and having only a vague idea of where to put your foot and hand next.

With the **Happiness Upgrade** method, it's easy to harness the mood-boosting power of small actions.

Ready to try giving yourself a **Happiness Upgrade** right now to see how it works? Read on…

How to give yourself a Happiness Upgrade

The **Happiness Upgrade** method is a simple technique that involves three key steps:

Step 1. Imagine a "happiness scale" that spans from 1 to 10.

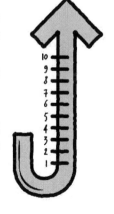

The bottom of the scale is **1**, which is the lowest your mood gets. This is when you're overwhelmed with anger, anxiety, despair, grief, hopelessness, regret, sadness, stress or another unwanted negative emotion.

The top of the scale is **10**, which is the highest your mood gets. This is when you're experiencing the kind of positivity that fills you with euphoric joy.

Step 2. Figure out where you are on this happiness scale now.

Think about what kind of mood you're experiencing this very moment.

Are you at a **1** where you're feeling overwhelmed with sadness, regret or another negative emotion?

Are you somewhere in the middle, such as a **5**, where you're not terribly sad, but not blissful either? Maybe you're bored, distracted or just going through the motions?

Are you at a **9** where you're almost at your absolute happiest?

Take your emotional temperature and try to determine where you fall on the happiness scale. There is no right or wrong answer. Base it on how you feel. Keep in mind that the happiness scale is subjective, so one person's **5** might be another person's **7**.

Step 3. Ask yourself: "What is an easy, healthy, positive action I can take right now to move myself up one step on the happiness scale?"

This is where your imagination comes in handy. Use it to think of simple ways you could give yourself a tiny mood boost. These could be self-care techniques (such as meditating or taking a break), hobbies (such as playing an instrument or painting), getting more comfortable (for example, by putting a pillow on your chair or changing the thermostat temperature) or other easy pick-me-ups.

Then, select one small action to do right now.

To understand how you can use this technique, here are a few examples:

Are you going from a bottomed-out 1 to a slightly better 2? Think of one small action you can take that would lessen your emotional pain just a bit, giving you enough relief from your overwhelming feelings to bring you up one step on the happiness scale. Maybe it's going outside to breathe in fresh air, making yourself a soothing cup of tea, wrapping yourself in a comforting throw blanket or visiting a website with cute animals to get a smile.

Are you going from an average 5 to a slightly more sparkly 6? Think about what you could easily do to boost your mood just a smidgen. For instance, you could give yourself a rejuvenating head massage, dab on a scent you enjoy or take a few minutes to shoot some hoops in your yard.

Going from a joyous 9 to a superlative 10? One great benefit of the **Happiness Upgrade** is that it helps you make pleasurable experiences even more enjoyable. That's because it spurs you to look for ways to intensify the activity in a way you may not have considered. For example, you could invite neighbors over to share a cake you just baked or turn on music while doing a favorite hobby.

Once you've moved yourself up one step on your **Happiness Upgrade** scale, pause and enjoy it. Savor the moment of pleasure, peace, calm, lower stress or sense of control. Then, consider if you want to stay where you are on the scale or move yourself up one more notch. If you want to go up one more, simply repeat these steps.

Bonus tips

To ensure your **Happiness Upgrade** is effective...

- **Avoid thinking big.** The most effective approach when using the **Happiness Upgrade** method is to aim for a mood-boosting action that's small, such as turning on music, brewing a cup of tea or opening a window to let in fresh air, since they're easy and can be done right now. Planning big, elaborate goals as your mood-booster, such as switching careers or moving to a new town, takes far more time and effort, which means you won't reap the emotional benefits for a long while.

- **Focus on moving up one step at a time.** When giving yourself a **Happiness Upgrade**, aim to move up just one step on your inner happiness scale, for example, from a **4** to a **5**. If you try leapfrogging up several steps at once, for example, going from a **4** to a **7**, you may get discouraged if it doesn't work. The one-step-at-a-time approach is more achievable. And, every time it works, you'll be motivated to try it again and again, which will eventually bring you up to where you want to be on your happiness scale.

- **Select actions that only move your mood in a *positive* direction**. This means skipping actions that could potentially lead to health issues or harmful negativity, for example, avoid turning to drugs or alcohol, food if you have food issues, spending money if you have money issues and taking a risk if you have impulse control issues. These kinds of actions may make you feel good in the moment, but they can send your mood spiraling down your happiness scale after the initial buzz wears off. By choosing activities that are uplifting, healthy and appropriate for you, you'll ensure you head in an upward direction.

- **Customize your happiness scale if desired.** Do you prefer to have a more finely-tuned numerical system, for example, by using fractions to know when you're rising from a **6** to a **6.5** or falling from an **8** to a **7.5**? Go ahead and use a happiness scale that works for you. As long as it helps you keep track of your mood in moment, it's the right scale for you.

Chapter 3:
How the Happiness Upgrade Can Help You

Before you continue reading this chapter, take a moment to pause and imagine a scene. Think back to a recent time when you were stressed, frustrated, annoyed or unhappy another way. For example, did you get an unexpected bill in the mail? Did someone not appreciate a favor you did for them? Were you overwhelmed from caring for a child or adult in need?

Try to remember how long the negative mood from the situation lasted. Did it ruin your lunch? Sour your whole day? Drag on even longer?

Now picture an imaginary button you could press that would pause that negative mood, then push you in a more positive direction so you felt just a little better. This way, you could cope with the stress of that unexpected bill. You could stop churning over the resentment of someone not appreciating your time and effort. You could feel less depleted while taking care of someone else.

This is how the **Happiness Upgrade** method can help you in everyday life.

What the Happiness Upgrade gives you

The **Happiness Upgrade** method doesn't promise euphoric joy in an instant. Or a day. Or even a week. It won't plaster a smile on your face 24/7 or insist you smile when you're not feeling it. It can't instantly fix stressful jobs, mend unhappy relationships or cure illnesses. It won't magically make sadness disappear or ask you to mask negative emotions.

Instead, the **Happiness Upgrade** method is a practical tool you can use to pause a negative mood, preventing it from falling further. And, it can change the direction of your mood so that instead of going down, it moves upward in a more positive path.

The **Happiness Upgrade** method delivers this by showing you how to harness the power of making small moves to improve your mood. It all starts with imagining a happiness scale of **1** to **10**, where **1** is the lowest mood and **10** is the highest. First, you rank where your current mood falls on this scale. Then, you ask yourself one simple question: **"What is an easy, healthy, positive action I can take right now to move myself up one step on the happiness scale?"**

This tiny nudge upward is a more powerful tool than it may at first seem. That's because this one small step up can...

- Pause a negative mood, preventing a downward spiral into an even worse mood
- Spur an upward spiral into a better mood
- Make challenging situations, people or moments easier to handle, reducing stress
- Inspire you to discover quick, easy methods that help you cope with life's challenges, boosting resilience
- Enhance the pleasure you get from positive experiences, making them even more joy-inducing

On top of all this, the **Happiness Upgrade** method is easy to use every day. That's because it...

- Works in seconds and can be used virtually anywhere, anytime
- Is small enough to be easy to do, yet powerful enough to impact your mood
- Can lead you to rising one more step up the happiness scale, then another, so you continue your upward spiral, boosting your mood even higher

The 5 secrets of the Happiness Upgrade

The **Happiness Upgrade** method seems simple enough: Imagine a happiness scale of **1** to **10**. Rate where you are on the scale.

Then, do one simple act to bring yourself one step higher on that scale.

But, behind this simple method are five secrets that explain why it works so well. They are:

Secret #1. You're recognizing when it's time for self-care.

In a typical day, how many times do you do something specifically for self-care, for example, give yourself a rejuvenating break by stepping outdoors, rub moisturizer onto dry hands, place a pillow behind an aching back, adjust the thermostat to a more comfortable temperature, pour yourself a refreshing glass of water, open a window to let in a cool breeze, have fun by turning on your favorite music, block out chatter with noise canceling headphones or take a few moments to calm yourself with slow, deep breaths? Probably fewer than you'd like or need.

It makes sense though since we rarely add self-care to our to-do list. As a result, it's easy to get swept up in tasks, responsibilities, obligations, errands, routines, distractions, problems and interruptions and forget to carve out a few moments to take care of ourselves.

The **Happiness Upgrade** method fixes this by making it easy to recognize when it's time for self-care. That's because the **1** to **10** happiness scale gives you a tool to rate how you feel at any given moment. This means when you notice your mood start to dip, you can picture this decline in mood on a numerical scale, for example, going from a **6** to a **5**. Thinking about self-care treatments in terms of having a concrete result—going up one number on your happiness scale, for example, from a **5** back up to a **6**—can be the motivation you need to give yourself a **Happiness Upgrade**.

Secret #2. You're aiming for a small, easy mood-booster that's doable.

Often, we daydream of big changes that could make us a whole lot happier, say, moving to a new town, saving enough money to buy a home, changing careers, going back to school, taking a vacation and finding a romantic partner. While it's certainly worth having big goals that could bring us intense joy, they can take a lot of time, effort and resources, which means waiting weeks, months or even years for more joyful days to come.

Unfortunately, there are also plenty of times when there's nothing we can do to change difficult circumstances no matter how hard we try, for example, because we're taking care of an ailing parent or living in a certain town for our job. So, if there isn't even an option of wishful daydreams becoming reality, then you're stuck waiting for more joyful days that never arrive.

The **Happiness Upgrade** takes a different approach to boosting mood. It focuses on creating small moments of joy in your *current everyday life*. This way, you don't have to wait to feel better until some distant point in the future. By pushing up your mood just one step on a happiness scale, you feel better right this minute.

Sure, the mood boost you get from a **Happiness Upgrade** likely won't be as euphoric as moving to a new town or changing careers. Yet, that little boost in good feelings can be enough to help you cope with a stressful situation or add more sparkle to a humdrum day, making today better.

Even more importantly, aiming to do a small, easy mood-booster makes you more likely to take action to feel happier. That's because doing something that brings you up one small step feels like an achievable goal that you can do virtually anywhere, anytime. As a result, you actually do it.

Secret #3. You're savoring the slight boost in mood.

If someone asked you to write down all the negative things that happened in your day and all the positive things that happened in your day, chances are, your list of negatives would be longer than the positives. Like a *lot* longer.

That's simply how humans are wired. The brain remembers stressful, angry and frightening experiences more vividly than happy moments as a way to keep you alive. After all, if you recall unpleasant encounters more clearly, such as a venomous snake slithering into your path, you'll be more likely to take safety precautions in the future, for example, by avoiding the area where you saw the scary snake.[1]

The problem is that this means memories of negative events that happen throughout a typical day (for example, realizing you forgot your wallet at home while already in the check-out line at the supermarket) can hang like a heavy cloud over you, souring your mood long after the event has passed.

Fortunately, the **Happiness Upgrade** method helps you balance these daily negatives by making the positives stand out more vibrantly. That's because it trains you to gauge where you are on your inner happiness scale, then notice as you move up a step to a slightly better mood. As a result, you're more aware of when your mood climbs. You feel it, for example, you might observe that there's less tension in your muscles or your heart rate has gone down. You know exactly what spurred the change—the **Happiness Upgrade** you gave yourself. You even rank it as a number on your happiness scale, say, going up from a **6** to a **7**. The positive bump in mood doesn't just flit by you unnoticed.

All this extra attention to moments of joy in your day means that you'll remember the **Happiness Upgrades** you gave yourself and how you felt better after you did them. And, when you look back on your day, sure, you'll still recall the emotional dings you got, but you'll also recall the emotional lifts you experienced more vividly, too.

Secret #4. You're realizing when you're already happy.

The **Happiness Upgrade** method's main purpose is to pause unwanted negative moods, such as sadness and frustration, and move your mood in a positive direction.

However, there's another benefit of using this technique: It enables you to recognize when you're *already happy*. For example, maybe your mood is brimming while you're taking a walk on a beautiful day or doing a favorite hobby. Gauging your good moods on the happiness scale of **1** to **10** gives you the tool to notice when your happiness level is at a high **7**, **8**, **9** or maybe even a **10**.

Acknowledging when your mood is already soaring is important for two key reasons: The first is that this awareness helps you savor joyful moments, making them more vibrant and memorable.

The second reason is that you can use the **Happiness Upgrade** to make this joyful moment even *more* mood-enhancing. That's because you can apply the same **Happiness Upgrade** principle that boosts your mood when it's low to boost your mood even higher when it's already elevated.

All it takes is thinking of one small, easy action that would make the experience more pleasurable. For example, during your walk outdoors, you could take a photo of a beautiful bird you pass. Or, you could create a music playlist that you listen to specifically while you do your favorite hobby. By nudging yourself up one more step on the happiness scale while you're already happy, you make the positive experience feel even more rewarding.

Secret #5. You're training yourself to make Happiness Upgrades a habit.

The **1** to **10** happiness scale that you use with the **Happiness Upgrade** method has many benefits. It...

- **Gives you something concrete to focus on.** It's easier to think of a mood-booster that's small and doable when you can picture it bringing you up one step on a happiness scale.
- **Makes you aware of when your mood has risen slightly.** By thinking about when you've moved up one step on your happiness scale, you get to savor that slight mood boost, which helps you appreciate it more.
- **Instills a sense of accomplishment.** When you realize that the **Happiness Upgrade** you gave yourself moved your mood up one step, it turns it into a goal that you've achieved. This gives you a moment where you have a

sense of control in a world where we often have little control. This, in itself, is a key factor in improving mood.

- **Strengthens the memory of when you gave yourself a Happiness Upgrade.** Imagining your mood as it moves up one step on your happiness scale makes it stand out in your mind at the end of the day. This has an important benefit: It makes it easier to look back on your day and spot times when you tend to need a **Happiness Upgrade** the most, for example, on the way to work or school. This means you can plan ahead to have **Happiness Upgrades** ready. For instance, you might create a special music playlist that you can listen to while commuting.

- **Helps determine which Happiness Upgrades that you tried worked best.** For example, maybe you discovered that stepping outdoors for a minute was more effective at boosting your mood than pouring yourself a cold glass of water. Or, perhaps you found that watching a funny YouTube video was easier to do than going outdoors. Once you pinpoint the **Happiness Upgrades** that work best for you (and using the journal in this book helps you do this), you can save time and lift good feelings more quickly and effectively.

And, there's one more important benefit of using the **1** to **10** inner happiness scale: You're training yourself to make **Happiness Upgrades** a regular habit. For instance, you may notice frustration rise as you're standing in a long line at a store or while stuck in traffic on the way to an appointment. Then, you automatically realize there's something easy you can do in that moment to nudge up your mood.

Once you reach this point, it means you're more finely tuned to your thoughts and feelings. You intuitively know when you need to pause unwanted negativity and how to lift positivity with small acts.

So, after using the happiness scale a while, perhaps three months, six months or a year, you may find you don't need to rely on it as a barometer of your mood every time to give yourself a

Happiness Upgrade. You can simply take a small mood-boosting action without thinking about where you are on a **1** to **10** scale.

However, if you notice that you're forgetting to take time for self-care or are spiraling down into longer, more intense negative moods, re-adopt the **1** to **10** happiness scale for a tune-up.

Bonus benefits of a Happiness Upgrade

Giving yourself a **Happiness Upgrade** improves your mood in the moment. Plus, it can have beneficial impacts on your future and health. That's because when your mood improves a little, you might get motivated to take other actions that lead to feeling more fulfilled or supported, making your life better. Some examples: You may join a social group, enroll in school, sign up for job training, visit a healthcare provider, start an exercise routine, eat nutritious foods or reach out to loved ones more often. Numerous studies show that happier people are more likely to adopt these kinds of good-for-you habits because they have more optimism about the future, making these actions feel like worthwhile investments.[2]

No need to fake a smile

The **Happiness Upgrade** method can add more joyful moments to your day and even make your overall life better. However, it can't eliminate all negative emotions. And that's a *good* thing. That's because some uncomfortable feelings are useful and necessary. For instance, regret helps you learn from mistakes. Grief is a natural part of processing a loss. Anger helps you cope with an injustice. And stress helps you clarify when a situation needs to be changed.

The **Happiness Upgrade** method isn't about fostering "toxic positivity", where you try to keep a smile on your face while ignoring the world crashing around you. It's normal and healthy to experience a full spectrum of emotions in response to the ups and downs of life.

But, the **Happiness Upgrade** can help reduce "toxic negativity", which are emotions that can have a damaging effect, such as feeling overwhelmed, deep sadness, high stress and rumination. Left unchecked, these feelings can lead to depression, anxiety, burnout, heart problems and other troublesome issues, or worsen pre-existing issues like these.

The purpose of the **Happiness Upgrade** method is to find healthy, positive ways to pivot away from toxic negativity by coping in the moment when unhealthy negative feelings arise. It's about remembering to dole out self-care in small, bite-sized amounts when you need them as a way to pause emotional pain, and to help lift your mood just a little. It also helps you become more aware of joyful times in your life, so you can savor them, and even enhance them.

Chapter 4:
Make the Happiness Upgrade Method Work Even Better

There's a simple way to make the **Happiness Upgrade** method work more easily and powerfully: Over the course of a week, use the **1** to **10** happiness scale to assess your average mood when things aren't going especially wrong or especially right. When life is just humming along at an even keel, ask yourself, **"Where does my mood usually fall on my inner happiness scale?"** Is it a **4**, **5**, **6**, **7** or another number? This is your *default happiness level*— the general mood you feel on a typical, ordinary day.

Your default happiness level is unique to you, so it will be different from someone else's. For example, my default happiness level is a quiet, yet satisfied **6**. My husband, Douglas, idles at a slightly more extroverted and sunnier **7**.

The point of a default happiness level

Knowing your default happiness level gives you a concrete number so you can measure your mood quickly and easily. You'll know if you're a-okay, if you're dropping down or if you're rising up.

For example, when I'm at a **6**, my personal default happiness level, it gives me a sense of comfort and serenity. I know I'm in balance.

When I drop down to a **5**, it means something frustrating may have happened or I may be experiencing higher stress. This is when I realize I need to use one of my favorite **Happiness Upgrades** to stall the downward trend.

When I rise to a **7** on my happiness scale, I know something good has happened or I've given myself a **Happiness Upgrade**. I become more aware of the extra boost in joy and, as a result, appreciate it more.

There may be times when circumstances push your mood down so far that you're unable to bring yourself all the way back up to your default happiness level. Some examples might include when a loved one is ill, your business is in jeopardy or you were let go from your job.

When challenges are severe like this, you don't have to try to bring yourself all the way back up to your default happiness level since it may not be possible. Instead, focus on giving yourself a **Happiness Upgrade** to pause the downward trend in mood and move your emotions upward in a more positive direction. In these instances, you can use your default happiness number to recognize when you're making progress.

Your default happiness can change

There is a popular theory in psychology called "set-point happiness" that's been around since the 1970s. When first introduced, researchers theorized that your inner happiness level is generally stable and based primarily on genetic factors and personality traits that are determined early on in your life. Sure, you'll have your ups and downs. For example, you could win lots of cash in a lottery or lose a loved one to cancer. However, according to this theory, you eventually return to your original "set point" of happiness. For instance, you get used to having extra money from your lottery winnings, so it's no longer as rewarding. And, you cope with your grief and loss, so eventually it's not as painful. You ultimately adapt to your life's circumstances. So, no matter what happens to you—good or bad—your general happiness level is predestined.[1]

However, other scientists believed this set-point happiness theory was too restrictive. After all, if you can't increase your typical happiness level, why even try? And, in fact, they discovered that you *can* improve your set-point happiness level. When analyzing the results of a 25-year survey of more than 60,000 people in Germany, investigators found that personal choices you make, such as being altruistic, maintaining a work/life balance, exercising and socializing, can raise your set-point happiness.[2] So, as it turns out, you aren't trapped into one happiness level by genetics and personality traits.

What does this mean for you? After you discover your default happiness level by using the **Happiness Upgrade** method for a week or so, you may find that your default happiness number could possibly be different a few months from now or next year or a few years down the road. This could be due to a multitude of reasons. For example, if you develop a new challenging health condition that interferes with everyday life, your default happiness level could possibly fall. Or, if symptoms of a health issue you've been facing ease up, your default happiness level could potentially rise.

Your default happiness level is a tool

You've already read that the **Happiness Upgrade** method's **1** to **10** happiness scale is a useful tool that helps you realize when your mood is rising or falling in the moment. Well, your default happiness level is also a useful tool: It shows you when your overall mood is at a level where you're comfortable and in balance, and it makes it easier to recognize if this default happiness level is rising or falling over a long period.

Being aware of changes in your default happiness level is helpful in itself. For instance, it can be a sign that it's time to talk with a healthcare provider if you feel you're at risk of depression because your default happiness level is getting precariously low, say, you dropped from a **6** to a **3**. Or, it can help you appreciate how your life is getting better because you notice your default happiness number has risen, say from a **5** to a **6**.

Chapter 5:
How You Can Use the Happiness Upgrade

The **Happiness Upgrade** method can give you a mood boost in a wide variety of situations. Following are some examples, plus ways I've used the **Happiness Upgrade** method in my own life and how other folks have used it in theirs.

You can give yourself a **Happiness Upgrade** to...

Cope with stressful days

No matter how hard we try to avoid stress, most of us end up experiencing tense moments at some point. For instance, you may receive an unexpected bill, get into a fender bender or lose your wallet. Or, you may be dealing with chronic stress due to difficulties at work, challenges at home or a never-ending to-do list.

Giving yourself a **Happiness Upgrade** on stressful days gives you a bit of a breather that helps replenish some of your mental and physical resources. This way, you can keep going despite the tension.

> *"I teach special education for kindergarten and first grade. This school year has been hell. I had no instructional aide and limited support staff. There were climbing numbers of students: It started with 5 kids and shot up to 14. And, the kids were so far behind in every developmental area due to shutdowns. Ugh! I did not want to go into that classroom every day.*
>
> *"I had already planned a leave of absence, but even counting down the days did not help me see the light at the end of the tunnel. So, I tried the **Happiness Upgrade** method. For example, when I was tired of struggling with student behaviors all day, I would let us all take a break and dance to a song*

or sit and read to them. Sometimes, I would just break out into song while walking them to the playground or lunch or while they were coming into the classroom from recess. I know it sounds like a no-brainer, but we have a tight teaching schedule that does not allow for fun.

"The **Happiness Upgrades** *were a perfect way to keep my sanity, and the students felt the same, I'm sure. We got to blow off some steam and enjoy each other's company."*
—*Amy B., Long Beach, California, United States*

"I knew I had a lot to do today. The stress was making its presence known, so I acknowledged it and looked around to see what might boost my mood. In front of me was the end of the morning sunrise, beautiful as ever. So, I took a breath, self-reflected, accepted and paused to see what I could do to help myself. Just a moment of beauty and a deep breath helped move me forward and my mood upward. And, it happened because I was thinking of how to upgrade my happiness. It's easy to let our body rule us, but in reality, we can learn to help ourselves and move our feelings to a better place with small steps like the **Happiness Upgrade.**"
—*Paula G., Ann Arbor, Michigan, United States*

"It was a tough day. My oldest kid was sick and couldn't go to school. My youngest is home, too, because he's high-risk and the recent spike in COVID-19 cases means he has to take extra precautions, so he's feeling lonely. I couldn't go to work and I've got other staff out at my school, so they're short-handed. On top of that, I've got to pack the house to move. It was just a really stressful day.

"So, I used the **Happiness Upgrade** *method today to bring up my mood. I decided we should all*

have a break. I told the kids they could watch TV for 20 minutes while they let Mom do her thing. During that time, I read an inspirational story a friend sent me and burned a blueberry-scented candle. After that, I was much calmer and more focused. I was able to jump back into my day and get going. It was exactly what I needed."
—*Jama F., Charlotte, North Carolina, United States*

"Over the course of about two weeks, I've had many stressful moments and moments of rumination I'd get caught up in. I'd find myself snapping at my husband or cringing when I'd hear the ding of a work message. In full disclosure, I'm dealing with major stressors: I broke my foot, moved cross-country over the holidays and am working extra hours while sleeping on an air mattress for three weeks. I felt like a squatter in my new home instead of the owner while the moving company just kept giving us excuses as to why our furniture was late.

*"When I felt myself getting irritated or cranky, I'd use the **Happiness Upgrade** method like I was hitting a Happiness Button, for example, when I saw my credit card was charged $10K by the moving company when I knew the truck hadn't left its origin. I felt my anxiety rising and, in my efforts to stay calm and centered, I visualized that button, and even drew a rough version of it in my notebook (looks more like a top hat…I'm not the best artist!) and pressed the paper sketch with my finger. This made me laugh at myself and then I rode that glimmer of feeling better to a memory of a particularly restful and magical time I had last summer sitting on the dock of a crystal-clear lake in Maine, eavesdropping on the sounds of nature and watching the dragonflies flit about while I sipped my coffee.*

"While I was still upset at the situation, I really did feel calmer and grateful for all the blessings I've enjoyed."
—Mickie C., Gig Harbor, Washington, United States

Handle circumstances that you can't control

You can use the **Happiness Upgrade** method to make it easier to cope with difficult situations that you have little control over, can't leave or can't change. Some examples: When you're taking care of an adult with dementia, in charge of rambunctious toddlers while battling a bad cold, in the waiting room of a hospital where a loved one is being treated or receiving hospital treatment yourself.

Finding a way to give yourself a bit of self-care in these highly challenging moments can help you feel a little more in control at a time when you may feel powerless. This can be enough to give you a small mood boost despite the difficult circumstances, which can then make you more resilient.

*"In 2015, I was in the hospital for a spinal fusion surgery, which is where two vertebrae in your back are fused together by attaching metal rods to them. As I lay in my hospital bed after surgery, I was in intense pain. I was also frustrated at being unable to move due to the long incision in my back held together with staples and the numerous machines that were hooked up all over my body. On a happiness scale, for me this moment was most certainly a low **2**.*

*"I was desperate to give myself a **Happiness Upgrade** so I could feel just a little brighter. Looking around the room, I assessed my options. It was a tiny, cramped space with a TV hung far away that got four channels, none of them clearly. Then, I noticed the closed window shades. I asked my husband to open them. There was a disappointing view of the*

35

back of a drab cement building outside. However, the sun was still able to peek over the concrete walls and reach my face.

"I focused all my attention on the sun's bright rays and how they warmed my cheeks. Despite my post-operative pain and frustration at being immobilized, this simple act was able to give me the slight lift in spirits I desperately needed, bringing me up one step to a 3 on my inner happiness scale.

"Years later, I still vividly recall how the sparkling sunlight and gentle warmth on my skin made me feel just a little better at one of my most difficult moments."
—Gabrielle Lichterman

Get past frustration

Annoyances have a way of popping out of the blue, threatening to spoil a perfectly good day. For example, an event you were looking forward to for weeks gets canceled at the last minute. You get half-way through making a recipe and realize you're missing a key ingredient and the grocery stores are now closed. Or, maybe you hit traffic, making you late for a meeting.

Whenever frustration rises in situations like these, you can use the **Happiness Upgrade** method to pause the downward negative spiral and bring your mood back up.

*"I used the **Happiness Upgrade** method while sitting in traffic. I'm used to sitting in Los Angeles traffic, however, when it's paired with running late for something, I can get so upset! Instead of hitting the steering wheel and swearing, or even crying, I forced myself to take some slow deep breaths and cranked up the music. It also helped to remind me about the end result of being a little late: Was it really going to ruin my life? No, I'd just be a little late."*
—Amy B., Long Beach, California, United States

Calm anxiety

It's normal to worry about something that could possibly happen in the future or something that most certainly is going to occur soon, for example, a medical procedure or the outcome of an important school exam. However, when you're consumed with worry or you're nervous about outcomes that have an extremely low likelihood of happening, this becomes anxiety, a condition that fills you with heightened dread and makes it difficult to turn off troubling thoughts of everything that could possibly go wrong.

In times like these, you can use the **Happiness Upgrade** method to distract yourself from nervous thoughts. This can help pause anxiousness so you don't keep churning over worst-case scenarios. A **Happiness Upgrade** can also reduce the impact of anxiety on your body, for example, it can help you relax tense muscles and ease a queasy stomach.

> *"I had to have oral surgery. Like most folks, on the day before the appointment I became increasingly worried about pain, needles and complications. I've had terrible dental experiences in the past and, even though this procedure was with a different surgeon who I liked, all those negative memories came flooding back and kept feeding my anxiety.*
>
> *"I could feel my happiness level drop from a typical-for-me 6 to a 5. And, I could tell that as my worry went on, my happiness level was going to continue to plunge. If that happened, I knew I would end up with a migraine and stomachache, making my day even more miserable.*
>
> *"So, I turned to one of my favorite **Happiness Upgrades** that I use when my anxiety rises: cleaning. I get so absorbed in scrubbing, soaping and organizing that I can almost forget my worries.*
>
> *"I grabbed my cleaning bucket, headed to the bathroom and got to work. In just a few minutes, this **Happiness Upgrade** tactic distracted my worried*

*thoughts, pausing me at a **5**. It wasn't enough to bring me back up to my default happiness level of **6**. (Only being told I wouldn't need surgery would do that!) However, I was able to halt the downward trend and dodge a headache and stomach pain."*
—Gabrielle Lichterman

Recover from setbacks

Life rarely delivers win after win after win. More typically, we experience wins, then losses, then more wins, then more losses. These kinds of setbacks can touch virtually every part of your life: You may get accepted into your first-pick university, but then not qualify for enough financial aid to attend. You may find your perfect job, but it's in a city that's too far to commute to. You may find your dream home, but then someone else buys it.

Sometimes, it's easy to shake off these disappointments and move on. Other times, the letdowns can spur a downward spiral of sadness or regret. This is when giving yourself a **Happiness Upgrade** can help by pausing the negativity and turning your mood in a positive direction.

"I was recently riding in the car with my husband and kids and began to feel blue. We're looking for a house and have been disappointed with several offers that had fallen through. On top of that, I've been stressed due to my job as a director of a school in the middle of a pandemic while pregnant. So, I thought this is a good time to rank where I am on my happiness scale and do one simple thing to bring me up one step.

"That's when I came up with a plan to take 20 minutes for myself once we got home to enjoy a long shower because I knew that this kind of self-care would make me feel better. But, then I instantly got a boost in mood just anticipating that I was going to do that for myself!"
—Jama F., Charlotte, North Carolina, United States

Solve a problem

Sometimes, a **Happiness Upgrade** means coming up with a solution for a nagging problem you've been facing so your life is just a little easier. This could include anything, such as fixing a wobbly table leg, finding a stylist who specializes in your type of hair or figuring out a way to make a healthy swap in your diet.

"I had to give up my beloved daily black tea because my blood pressure was climbing and caffeine can make it worse. Unfortunately, not only did I rely on tea for a morning pick-me-up, but brewing a fresh cup was one of my favorite **Happiness Upgrades**. *I loved the ritual as much as the caffeinated kick. So, I was really disappointed.*

*"The first couple of weeks without tea were not easy. I was tired and cranky from caffeine withdrawal, which was dragging my default happiness level down from a **6** to a **5**. And, I no longer had that lovely tea-brewing* **Happiness Upgrade** *break to look forward to for a mood bump.*

"So, I thought about a new way to give myself a daily **Happiness Upgrade** *that would replace my tea. Then, it hit me: dark cocoa. It's chock full of flavonoids that lower blood pressure by widening blood vessels. Plus, it has its own natural stimulant, theobromine, which would work like caffeine to rev energy. It seemed like the perfect substitute.*

"I got a box of dark cocoa powder and made a cup from scratch. It was scrumptious and filled me with all the energy I was craving—while helping to lower my blood pressure. On top of that, it's fun to make. Now when I wake up, I instantly think of the delicious chocolately **Happiness Upgrade** *that awaits me and can't wait to get out of bed. Honestly, I wish I'd switched sooner!"*
—Gabrielle Lichterman

Reset your mood

In this go-go-go world, it's easy to forget to that your body isn't a go-go-go machine. It gets physically tired. It gets mentally overwhelmed. When this happens to you, the **Happiness Upgrade** method can remind you to take a break. This way, you can fully unwind after a long, intense experience, for example, after you've traveled for hours or unloaded boxes during a big move. Or, you can use the **Happiness Upgrade** method to rejuvenate yourself in the middle of an exceptionally busy day, for example, on your wedding day, when you're attending a long conference or if you're hosting a family holiday.

> *"I had 20 family members over for Christmas day lunch, so I got a little overwhelmed. I sent myself to my bedroom and took slow deep breaths to bring me back to the now. I checked my happiness level and it was lower than my usual 7. I took a deep breath and focused on how happy all my family were, how easy we were all getting on and how wonderful my festive home was looking. I checked my happiness level and, no surprise, it was back to my comfort level."*
> —Tess F., Brisbane, Queensland, Australia

Motivate yourself

Ever find yourself procrastinating, for example, putting off working on a report, completing a project or simply doing the dishes? You can harness the power of the **Happiness Upgrade** method to push yourself by taking quick self-care mini-breaks throughout or promising yourself a mood-boosting activity once you've finished it.

> *"There are times when I'll open a book, article, news tab, cute kitten video, Zillow Gone Wild or whatever my favorite distraction is, then I set it aside and say to myself, 'As soon as you finish the task, it's*

*all yours.' Just the anticipation of getting to stop and take that break will activate an upgrade in happiness, so while I'm enjoying the fruits of my labor, I typically get yet another **Happiness Upgrade!**"*
—Paula G., Ann Arbor, Michigan, United States

Enhance a happy moment

The **Happiness Upgrade** method reminds you to focus on the positives you're experiencing and find ways to add to them so they're even better.

*"I was feeling good, telling jokes with my husband, and thought about the **Happiness Upgrade**. I thought, 'Okay, let's keep this going, Mickie.' I consciously recognized what a fun moment I was enjoying and rode that feeling like surfing a gentle ocean wave."*
—Mickie C., Gig Harbor, Washington, United States

Get a mood boost anytime

Whether you notice you're sliding down your happiness scale or you simply want a little more sparkle in your day, you can give yourself a **Happiness Upgrade** that kicks in right away.

*"At a time when I was at a **5**, I wanted to try to get to a **6** and I thought, 'What could I do that would change the feeling straight away?' I looked out of the window and watched the birds on the bird feeder. I felt better than one minute beforehand. I was present in that moment and recognized that my happiness level had increased. Usually this is something that would pass me by, but actually taking the time to be present and giving yourself a happiness score every so often helps so much."*
—Hannah S., Lincolnshire, United Kingdom

Chapter 6:
Happiness Upgrade Suggestions

Eager to give yourself a **Happiness Upgrade**, but not sure where to begin? Below are quick suggestions for a wide variety of **Happiness Upgrades** to inspire you. You'll find 52 more study-backed **Happiness Upgrade** recommendations in the 52-week journal that follows this chapter.

Happiness Upgrades that reduce stress:
- Take deep, slow breaths
- Listen to relaxing music
- Give yourself a soothing arm, foot or head massage
- Stretch your body
- Take a break outdoors or watch a nature video

Happiness Upgrades that make life a little easier, whether it's at home, work, school, on the go or at appointments:
- Keep healthy snacks nearby for times when you're hungry, but have little time to take a meal break
- Create music playlists of artists you enjoy that you can listen to while traveling, waiting in line, sitting in waiting rooms, having dental treatments, working or studying
- Put extras of items you might need when on the go in your car or tote bag, such as hand sanitizer, a necktie, hair ties, socks or bottles of water
- Place a waterproof notepad and pencil in your shower to write down great ideas so you don't forget them
- Stash hidden games or books for the kids in your car glovebox, home office or tote bag for emergency distractions

Happiness Upgrades that improve your environment:
- Burn a scented candle or incense
- Put on headphones to drown out noise
- Raise window shades to let in sunlight

- Open a window to let in fresh air
- Turn on a HEPA filter to reduce indoor allergens

Happiness Upgrades that improve every room of your home:
- Safely place a radio or music player in your bathroom to listen to as you bathe
- Drape a throw blanket over your couch to wrap yourself in as you read or watch TV
- Store a box of gourmet tea, coffee or cocoa in your kitchen so you'll always have it when you want a special treat
- Place a pair of warm socks by your bedside so you'll have them in an instant if it gets too cold in the middle of the night
- Keep a pair of comfy slippers by the front door so you can trade them for your outdoor shoes or work shoes as soon as you step inside

Happiness Upgrades that make you more physically comfortable:
- Take off tight garments, such as a bra, tie, uniform, shoes, or work clothes
- Change the room temperature by raising or lowering the thermostat, turning on a heater, air conditioner or fan, or opening or closing a window
- Add a pillow to your chair
- Treat physical pain (for example, by using a pain reliever for a headache or heat patch for menstrual cramps) rather than power through it
- Rub moisturizer onto dry skin or lip balm onto chapped lips

Happiness Upgrades that are comforting:
- Make yourself a cup of cocoa, coffee or tea
- Dab on your favorite fragrance
- Give yourself a soothing shoulder rub

- Read inspirational quotes
- Put on your comfiest clothes or pajamas

Happiness Upgrades that treat yourself:
- Take a long bath
- Read a chapter of a book or watch a TV show or movie
- Buy yourself a gift
- Prepare or order a special meal
- Relax on a front lawn, park bench, patio, porch or stoop

Happiness Upgrades that recharge body and brain:
- Lighten your to-do list
- Stop doing an activity you don't enjoy, isn't fulfilling or makes you feel bad
- Exit from a stressful situation or draining conversation
- Unplug from the news, social media or email
- Take a break from work or other responsibilities

Happiness Upgrades that make you feel healthier right now:
- Take a walk
- Garden
- Practice yoga, meditation or tai chi or stretch your body
- Treat yourself to a vegetable salad or whole fruit smoothie
- Drink water

Happiness Upgrades that help you cultivate self-compassion:
- Forgive yourself for a mistake or embarrassing slip-up
- Give yourself the same supportive advice you'd give to a friend or family member
- Remind yourself that it's okay to not be perfect
- Read an uplifting passage from an inspirational or spiritual book
- Thank yourself for your good traits, good deeds, good ideas or other positive qualities and acts

52-Week

Happiness
Upgrade

Journal

Date _Monday, January 14_

Happiness Upgrades	before	after
Took a short walk	4	5
Brewed a cup of tea	5	6
Put pillow on my chair	5	6

Happiness Upgrade Journal

Your 52-week journal is a tool to track the **Happiness Upgrades** you try. This is helpful because it...

- Reminds you to incorporate **Happiness Upgrades** into your daily life
- Gives you a record of **Happiness Upgrades** that work for you, which means when you need one quickly, your favorite options are right at your fingertips
- Enables you to pinpoint trouble spots where you regularly need a **Happiness Upgrade** so you can prepare ahead of time, for example, you may want to create a soothing music playlist that calms you when driving in heavy traffic

Happiness Upgrade journal instructions

Using your journal to keep a record of the **Happiness Upgrades** you try is easy:

- Read how to give yourself a **Happiness Upgrade** in Chapter 2.
- When you're ready, give yourself a **Happiness Upgrade**, for example, take a short walk, brew a cup of tea or put a pillow on your chair.
- Note your experience in your journal by writing the date and which **Happiness Upgrade** you used.
- Rank your mood on a happiness scale of **1** to **10** before and after the **Happiness Upgrade**.
- The goal is to go up one step on your inner happiness scale, for example rising from a **4** to a **5**. However, if you prefer, you can use a more finely-tuned

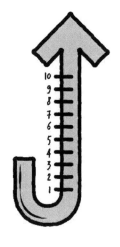

numerical system, for example, using fractions that indicate when you're rising from a **5** to a **5.5**.

- You may notice that your mood goes down or up as the day goes on due to a variety of circumstance you encounter. So, just note where you are on your happiness scale in the moment when you try a **Happiness Upgrade**.

Happiness Upgrade journal example:

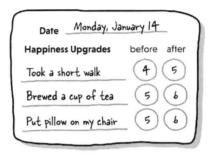

- Optional: Note your default happiness level, which is where your mood falls on your happiness scale on a typical day (learn more in Chapter 4).

52 Happiness Upgrades to try

Throughout your journal you'll find 52 study-backed **Happiness Upgrade** suggestions to try—one for each week of the year. In addition, you'll get a list of seven different ways to try each suggestion—one for each day of the week.

Feel free to follow these suggestions or use them as inspiration for creating your own.

Happiness Upgrade:
Look at Nature

For an easy **Happiness Upgrade**, gaze at birds, flowers, a pond or any other parts of nature. You'll feel uplifted within moments.[1] This effect occurs whether you look at a real-life nature scene (for instance, outside your window) or an image (say, on a computer screen).

Why it works

Researchers theorize that humans evolved to feel happy and at peace when viewing nature because it meant basic necessities (food, water and shelter) were likely nearby. Plus, the wonder and beauty of nature distract you from worries, which reduces stress. On top of that, nature reminds you that you're part of something much larger, which can give your life more meaning.

Happiness Upgrade suggestions:

1. Change your computer or phone wallpaper to a nature scene.
2. Hang a bird feeder or place a bird bath outside your window to attract robins, finches or other birdlife.
3. Switch an item you use every day (such as a mug) to one that is adorned with an image of an animal, mountain scene or other natural element.
4. Search online for pictures of beaches, forests, waterfalls or other outdoor settings.
5. Place a live potted plant where you can see it.
6. Put fresh-cut flowers in a vase.
7. Use your smartphone to take photos of nature that you like as you come across it, then take a peek at your pics whenever you need a **Happiness Upgrade**.

Happiness Upgrade Journal

*Give yourself a Happiness Upgrade, then note where you rank
on a happiness scale of 1 to 10 before and after.*

Date _____

Happiness Upgrades   before   after

_____ ◯ ◯

_____ ◯ ◯

_____ ◯ ◯

Date _____

Happiness Upgrades   before   after

_____ ◯ ◯

_____ ◯ ◯

_____ ◯ ◯

Date _____

Happiness Upgrades   before   after

_____ ◯ ◯

_____ ◯ ◯

_____ ◯ ◯

Date _____

Happiness Upgrades   before   after

_____ ◯ ◯

_____ ◯ ◯

_____ ◯ ◯

Date _____

Happiness Upgrades   before   after

_____ ◯ ◯

_____ ◯ ◯

_____ ◯ ◯

Date _____

Happiness Upgrades   before   after

_____ ◯ ◯

_____ ◯ ◯

_____ ◯ ◯

Date _____

Happiness Upgrades   before   after

_____ ◯ ◯

_____ ◯ ◯

_____ ◯ ◯

Default
Happiness Level

Happiness Upgrade:
Get Busy

Have some free time on your hands? For example, maybe you've discovered an opening in your day when you don't need to take care of work, the kids or chores? Or, perhaps you're on vacation? The idea of doing absolutely nothing may sound tempting, but you'll give yourself a mood-boosting **Happiness Upgrade** if you fill this time with an activity that keeps you mentally or physically active. That's the news from a study in the journal *Psychological Science* that found folks who keep busy doing virtually *anything* during their leisure-time are happier than those who do nothing at all.[1]

Why it works

Your brain thrives on activity, so you can become bored and restless when you're idle, which drags down your mood. By staying active, you keep your mind engaged, pushing up positivity.

Happiness Upgrade suggestions:

1. Enjoy a favorite hobby, such as baking, knitting, playing music, reading or woodworking.
2. Go for a walk, hop on a bike, ride a skateboard or put on your inline skates.
3. Organize an area of your home, office or workshop.
4. Call a friend to catch up.
5. Create art.
6. Play with your pet or tend to plants.
7. Chip away at a big project, such as writing a novel, coming up with a business plan or building a bookshelf.

Happiness Upgrade Journal

*Give yourself a Happiness Upgrade, then note where you rank
on a happiness scale of 1 to 10 before and after.*

Date _____

Happiness Upgrades   before   after

_____ ◯ ◯

_____ ◯ ◯

_____ ◯ ◯

Date _____

Happiness Upgrades   before   after

_____ ◯ ◯

_____ ◯ ◯

_____ ◯ ◯

Date _____

Happiness Upgrades   before   after

_____ ◯ ◯

_____ ◯ ◯

_____ ◯ ◯

Date _____

Happiness Upgrades   before   after

_____ ◯ ◯

_____ ◯ ◯

_____ ◯ ◯

Date _____

Happiness Upgrades   before   after

_____ ◯ ◯

_____ ◯ ◯

_____ ◯ ◯

Date _____

Happiness Upgrades   before   after

_____ ◯ ◯

_____ ◯ ◯

_____ ◯ ◯

Date _____

Happiness Upgrades   before   after

_____ ◯ ◯

_____ ◯ ◯

_____ ◯ ◯

Default
Happiness Level

Happiness Upgrade:
Try Something New

One way to get a **Happiness Upgrade** quickly is to do something you normally don't. You can pick an activity that's far outside your usual comfort zone, say, posting your first TikTok video. Or, you can choose an activity that varies just slightly from your everyday habits, such as getting lunch from a different food truck. Whatever you select, trying anything new will give you an instant spike in mood-lifting excitement.

Tip: Make it a habit to regularly have new experiences. Research in the journal *Nature Neuroscience* shows that folks who expose themselves to at least one new thing daily are happier than those following the same humdrum routine. And, those who fit the most variety into each day get the biggest surge in positivity of all.[1]

Why it works

Experiencing something new triggers the production of the feel-good neurotransmitter dopamine in brain, which gives you a rewarding sensation. Researchers suspect one key reason this pleasurable reaction to newness evolved in humans was to encourage us to travel to unfamiliar places to find food despite the fear of unknown threats.

Happiness Upgrade suggestions:

1. Talk with new people, for instance, chat with a stranger while in line at a store or join a social group.
2. Experiment with a different restaurant or recipe.
3. Travel somewhere unfamiliar or take a different route.
4. Be spontaneous, for example, pop into a shop or art gallery you've passed a hundred times, but never entered.
5. Try a sport, hobby or other activity you haven't done before.
6. Sign up for a class to learn something different.
7. Pick an event to attend from you local events calendar.

Happiness Upgrade Journal

*Give yourself a Happiness Upgrade, then note where you rank
on a happiness scale of 1 to 10 before and after.*

Date _____

Happiness Upgrades   before   after

_____   ○   ○

_____   ○   ○

_____   ○   ○

Date _____

Happiness Upgrades   before   after

_____   ○   ○

_____   ○   ○

_____   ○   ○

Date _____

Happiness Upgrades   before   after

_____   ○   ○

_____   ○   ○

_____   ○   ○

Date _____

Happiness Upgrades   before   after

_____   ○   ○

_____   ○   ○

_____   ○   ○

Date _____

Happiness Upgrades   before   after

_____   ○   ○

_____   ○   ○

_____   ○   ○

Date _____

Happiness Upgrades   before   after

_____   ○   ○

_____   ○   ○

_____   ○   ○

Date _____

Happiness Upgrades   before   after

_____   ○   ○

_____   ○   ○

_____   ○   ○

Default
Happiness Level

Happiness Upgrade:
Admire Art

When you're in need of a **Happiness Upgrade**, gaze at a drawing, painting, photograph, sculpture or other work of visual art that you personally find beautiful. Researchers out of University College London in the United Kingdom discovered that viewing artwork you enjoy gives you an instant bump in good feelings.[1]

Why it works

Using fMRI brain scans, the scientists found that looking at works of art you find appealing triggers greater blood flow to an area of the brain that spurs sensations of pleasure and reward (medial orbito-frontal cortex) and an area that's involved with warm, loving emotions (caudate nucleus), making them more active.

Happiness Upgrade suggestions:

1. Visit a museum or art gallery. Or, check out an exhibit being displayed in a school, café or retail store.
2. Look for free online art museum tours, for example, at Google.com/culturalinstitute.
3. Attend an art opening.
4. Head to a bookstore or library and leaf through books featuring your favorite visual artists.
5. Attend a craft fair or local outdoor art exhibit.
6. Bookmark websites of your favorite visual artists on your computer, phone or other device.
7. Create your own art and display it.

Happiness Upgrade Journal

*Give yourself a Happiness Upgrade, then note where you rank
on a happiness scale of 1 to 10 before and after.*

Date _____
Happiness Upgrades   before   after

Date _____
Happiness Upgrades   before   after

Date _____
Happiness Upgrades   before   after

Date _____
Happiness Upgrades   before   after

Date _____
Happiness Upgrades   before   after

Date _____
Happiness Upgrades   before   after

Date _____
Happiness Upgrades   before   after

Default
Happiness Level

Happiness Upgrade:
Change the Temperature

Take a moment to notice if you're a bit too warm or too chilly. If you are, give yourself a **Happiness Upgrade** by doing something that can help you get cooler or toastier.

Why it works

The human body is designed to function best at a comfortable temperature, which means that when it's a little out of that optimal zone—too hot or too cold—it can make you irritable. By doing what you can to move closer to your temperature sweet spot, you improve your mood.[1]

Happiness Upgrade suggestions:

1. Open a window or two to let in a fresh, cool breeze or let out stuffy warm air.
2. Adjust the thermostat or air conditioner.
3. Put on or take off a sweater or jacket.
4. Wrap yourself in a cozy blanket or scarf.
5. Warm up socks, pajamas or a blanket in the dryer or stick them in the refrigerator to chill them.
6. Turn on a fan.
7. Move to a different part of the room away from or closer to a fan, air conditioning vent or heater.

Happiness Upgrade Journal

Give yourself a Happiness Upgrade, then note where you rank on a happiness scale of 1 to 10 before and after.

Date _____
Happiness Upgrades   before   after
_____ ○ ○
_____ ○ ○
_____ ○ ○

Date _____
Happiness Upgrades   before   after
_____ ○ ○
_____ ○ ○
_____ ○ ○

Date _____
Happiness Upgrades   before   after
_____ ○ ○
_____ ○ ○
_____ ○ ○

Date _____
Happiness Upgrades   before   after
_____ ○ ○
_____ ○ ○
_____ ○ ○

Date _____
Happiness Upgrades   before   after
_____ ○ ○
_____ ○ ○
_____ ○ ○

Date _____
Happiness Upgrades   before   after
_____ ○ ○
_____ ○ ○
_____ ○ ○

Date _____
Happiness Upgrades   before   after
_____ ○ ○
_____ ○ ○
_____ ○ ○

Default Happiness Level

Happiness Upgrade:
Tend to a Garden

You can give yourself a **Happiness Upgrade** every time you tend to flowers, herbs or other greenery. No matter how big or small your garden or whether it's indoors or outdoors, nourishing plants is a study-proven way to push up positivity.

Why it works

Gardening boosts mood a variety of ways: When you dig into soil, you breathe in its "good" bacteria, *Mycobacterium vaccae*, which prompts the production of mood-lifting serotonin and curbs inflammation, helping to thwart the blues and anxiety.[1] Simply seeing live plants triggers happiness and relaxation possibly because the brain is wired to feel blissful in the presence of nature since it's a sign that food may be nearby.[2] Gardening also distracts you from worries, gives you an opportunity to chat with neighbors and prompts you to keep moving, which all increase good feelings and rein in stress.[3]

Happiness Upgrade suggestions:

1. Plant seeds for herbs that you use regularly in the kitchen or that will inspire you to try new recipes.
2. Create a vegetable garden or plant fruit trees.
3. Build a garden that attracts butterflies, bees or other wildlife.
4. Look for free flowers, plants, ornamental grasses, shrubs or trees being given away by neighbors.
5. Boost the health of existing potted plants by transferring them to larger pots that give their roots more room to spread.
6. Give the gift of potted greenery to others.
7. Make a garden specifically for your pets, such as a catnip corner for your cat and grassy patch for your dog.

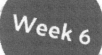

Happiness Upgrade Journal

Give yourself a Happiness Upgrade, then note where you rank on a happiness scale of 1 to 10 before and after.

Date _____

Happiness Upgrades   before   after

_____   ○   ○
_____   ○   ○
_____   ○   ○

Date _____

Happiness Upgrades   before   after

_____   ○   ○
_____   ○   ○
_____   ○   ○

Date _____

Happiness Upgrades   before   after

_____   ○   ○
_____   ○   ○
_____   ○   ○

Date _____

Happiness Upgrades   before   after

_____   ○   ○
_____   ○   ○
_____   ○   ○

Date _____

Happiness Upgrades   before   after

_____   ○   ○
_____   ○   ○
_____   ○   ○

Date _____

Happiness Upgrades   before   after

_____   ○   ○
_____   ○   ○
_____   ○   ○

Date _____

Happiness Upgrades   before   after

_____   ○   ○
_____   ○   ○
_____   ○   ○

Default Happiness Level

Happiness Upgrade:
Hug a Person or Pet

If you've got people or pets around, getting a **Happiness Upgrade** is as easy as giving them a warm hug.

Why it works

Gentle, welcome touch increases the production of the hormone oxytocin in the brain, which improves mood and makes you feel more trusting, closer and in tune with others. It also lowers the stress hormone cortisol, so you become more relaxed.[1]

Happiness Upgrade suggestions:

1. Ask your child, parent, partner or sibling for a hug.
2. Cuddle your cat, dog, hamster, horse or other "hug-friendly" pet.
3. Meet up with a friend who enjoys a good hug.
4. Volunteer to hug animals at shelters who are looking for new homes to help socialize them.
5. Volunteer to cuddle babies in hospitals who are undergoing care and need the extra nurturing to heal.
6. Offer a hug to an isolated neighbor who could use friendly company.
7. Extend a hug to someone who's been under a lot of stress and could use comforting.

Happiness Upgrade Journal

Give yourself a Happiness Upgrade, then note where you rank on a happiness scale of 1 to 10 before and after.

Date _____
Happiness Upgrades   before   after
_____ ○ ○
_____ ○ ○
_____ ○ ○

Date _____
Happiness Upgrades   before   after
_____ ○ ○
_____ ○ ○
_____ ○ ○

Date _____
Happiness Upgrades   before   after
_____ ○ ○
_____ ○ ○
_____ ○ ○

Date _____
Happiness Upgrades   before   after
_____ ○ ○
_____ ○ ○
_____ ○ ○

Date _____
Happiness Upgrades   before   after
_____ ○ ○
_____ ○ ○
_____ ○ ○

Date _____
Happiness Upgrades   before   after
_____ ○ ○
_____ ○ ○
_____ ○ ○

Date _____
Happiness Upgrades   before   after
_____ ○ ○
_____ ○ ○
_____ ○ ○

Default
Happiness Level

Happiness Upgrade:
Leave Work Behind

It can be tempting to answer more emails, make more calls, chip away more at a project, clean one more room or continue to work in other ways after your workday is supposed to be over or on days when you're not even scheduled to work. After all, you might feel like you're being productive if you keep going and going. However, you'll actually give yourself a **Happiness Upgrade** when you grant yourself permission to leave responsibilities behind once your workday is done.

Why it works

According to research led by Portland State University in Oregon, disconnecting from your to-dos during your nonwork time replenishes mental energy, which makes you happier and more satisfied with life.[1]

Happiness Upgrade suggestions:

1. Signal the end of your workday with a special ritual, such as texting a loved one or brewing yourself a cup of tea.
2. Once your worktime is over, physically walk away from your work area, say, stroll through the neighborhood or a park.
3. Go farther: Take a bike, bus, car or train to put a few miles between you and your workspace.
4. After work hours, immerse yourself in a book, hobby, video game or music.
5. Turn off digital notifications, shut down your computer, put away tools or disconnect from your workday another way.
6. During vacations or quality time with family, friends or pets, put non-essential work aside.
7. Use auto replies on email and other digital communications to let folks know you're out of touch for non-urgent reasons until the next workday begins.

Happiness Upgrade Journal

*Give yourself a Happiness Upgrade, then note where you rank
on a happiness scale of 1 to 10 before and after.*

Date _____
Happiness Upgrades   before   after
_____ ○ ○
_____ ○ ○
_____ ○ ○

Date _____
Happiness Upgrades   before   after
_____ ○ ○
_____ ○ ○
_____ ○ ○

Date _____
Happiness Upgrades   before   after
_____ ○ ○
_____ ○ ○
_____ ○ ○

Date _____
Happiness Upgrades   before   after
_____ ○ ○
_____ ○ ○
_____ ○ ○

Date _____
Happiness Upgrades   before   after
_____ ○ ○
_____ ○ ○
_____ ○ ○

Date _____
Happiness Upgrades   before   after
_____ ○ ○
_____ ○ ○
_____ ○ ○

Date _____
Happiness Upgrades   before   after
_____ ○ ○
_____ ○ ○
_____ ○ ○

Default
Happiness Level

Happiness Upgrade:
Listen to Music

For a **Happiness Upgrade** at home or on the go, turn on your favorite music, listen to tunes you haven't heard in a while or check out songs that are new. Any kind of music you enjoy will help you through a variety of situations, for example, when frustrated (say, when stuck in traffic), bored (like when waiting for an appointment) or stressed (such as when you're working on an important project). An added bonus: Music makes fun activities (such as creating art and taking a walk) even more enjoyable.

Why it works

Pleasurable music cues the release of dopamine, a neurotransmitter in the brain that gives you a rewarding, satisfying sensation similar to what you'd experience when kissing, eating delicious food or receiving money.[1]

Happiness Upgrade suggestions:

1. Carry a portable music player and earphones so you can listen to tunes while shopping, waiting for appointments, commuting or doing other activities on the go.
2. Turn on a radio in the car, at work or at home.
3. Assemble specific playlists for different activities, such as while working, studying, creating art or tackling chores.
4. Enjoy music while walking, running, lifting weights and doing other exercise.
5. Swap playlists with your friends and family.
6. Listen to covers of favorite songs performed by other musical artists to hear unique renditions.
7. Check out videos or audio recordings of live performances by your favorite musical artists.

Happiness Upgrade Journal

*Give yourself a Happiness Upgrade, then note where you rank
on a happiness scale of 1 to 10 before and after.*

Date _____
Happiness Upgrades   before   after
_____   ○   ○
_____   ○   ○
_____   ○   ○

Date _____
Happiness Upgrades   before   after
_____   ○   ○
_____   ○   ○
_____   ○   ○

Date _____
Happiness Upgrades   before   after
_____   ○   ○
_____   ○   ○
_____   ○   ○

Date _____
Happiness Upgrades   before   after
_____   ○   ○
_____   ○   ○
_____   ○   ○

Date _____
Happiness Upgrades   before   after
_____   ○   ○
_____   ○   ○
_____   ○   ○

Date _____
Happiness Upgrades   before   after
_____   ○   ○
_____   ○   ○
_____   ○   ○

Date _____
Happiness Upgrades   before   after
_____   ○   ○
_____   ○   ○
_____   ○   ○

Default
Happiness Level

Happiness Upgrade:
Post a Love Note

Give yourself a **Happiness Upgrade** by jotting down a few traits you love about yourself, such as your compassion, generosity, intelligence, loyalty or sense of humor. Then, post it somewhere you'll see it several times throughout your day.

Why it works

Being reminded of what makes you a wonderful person activates reward pathways in the brain, resulting in instant happiness, report researchers in the journal *Psychological Science*.[1]

Happiness Upgrade suggestions:

1. Place your note on your bathroom mirror, computer monitor, coffee mug or refrigerator.
2. Take a picture of your note, then use it as your wallpaper for an electronic device you use daily.
3. Tape a note to something you take care of every day, such as the pot of a flower you water or food container for a pet.
4. Slip your message into a drawer you frequently open.
5. Place your note next to your toothbrush.
6. Attach your note to a window you look out during the day.
7. Stick your note to your bedroom clock or lamp so it's the first thing you see when waking up and last thing you see before going to sleep.

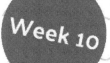

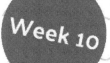
Week 10

Happiness Upgrade Journal

*Give yourself a Happiness Upgrade, then note where you rank
on a happiness scale of 1 to 10 before and after.*

Date _____
Happiness Upgrades   before   after

Date _____
Happiness Upgrades   before   after

Date _____
Happiness Upgrades   before   after

Date _____
Happiness Upgrades   before   after

Date _____
Happiness Upgrades   before   after

Date _____
Happiness Upgrades   before   after

Date _____
Happiness Upgrades   before   after

Default
Happiness Level

Happiness Upgrade:
Find More Members of Your Pack

Research shows that having a wide network of friends makes you more content with your life. But, you can give yourself a **Happiness Upgrade** and make this tip work even more effectively by joining groups that specifically reflect your personal interests, goals or beliefs. According to a study in the journal *PLOS ONE*, the more groups like these you belong to, the happier you become.[1]

Why it works

Being a member of groups filled with like-minded folks ratchets up self-esteem and gives you a greater feeling of support, connection and control in your life than simply having *any* kinds of friends.

Happiness Upgrade suggestions:

1. Join a group that gathers to do an activity together, for instance, a book club at a library, knitting circle at a crafts store, bicycle organization at a bike shop, bowling league at a bowling alley or walking club at a park.
2. Participate in religious, metaphysical, philosophical or spiritual study groups.
3. Team up with others to achieve good-for-you goals, such as reaching a healthy weight, quitting cigarettes, reducing stress or maintaining sobriety.
4. Look for professional organizations or networking functions.
5. Connect with folks who are following the same life path as you, such as activists, artists, entrepreneurs or volunteers.
6. Sign up for an in-person or online group class for a subject you enjoy.
7. Play games in person or online with other game enthusiasts, such as chess or Dungeons & Dragons.

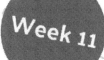

Happiness Upgrade Journal

Give yourself a Happiness Upgrade, then note where you rank on a happiness scale of 1 to 10 before and after.

Date _____		
Happiness Upgrades	before	after
_____	○	○
_____	○	○
_____	○	○

Date _____		
Happiness Upgrades	before	after
_____	○	○
_____	○	○
_____	○	○

Date _____		
Happiness Upgrades	before	after
_____	○	○
_____	○	○
_____	○	○

Date _____		
Happiness Upgrades	before	after
_____	○	○
_____	○	○
_____	○	○

Date _____		
Happiness Upgrades	before	after
_____	○	○
_____	○	○
_____	○	○

Date _____		
Happiness Upgrades	before	after
_____	○	○
_____	○	○
_____	○	○

Date _____		
Happiness Upgrades	before	after
_____	○	○
_____	○	○
_____	○	○

Default Happiness Level

Happiness Upgrade:
Chew Gum

Keep a pack of gum nearby, then when you need a **Happiness Upgrade**, stick a piece in your mouth and chew. You'll feel more upbeat, alert and focused within minutes, studies show.[1]

Why it works

Chewing sends oxygen-rich blood to the brain, increasing mental energy. An added bonus: If you're bothered by an ongoing loop of intrusive thoughts, movements that your mouth and jaw make as you chew may halt this rumination by short-circuiting the conversation going on inside your head, found researchers from the University of Reading in the United Kingdom.[2]

Happiness Upgrade suggestions:

1. Chew gum to decrease stress as you travel through heavy traffic, detours or unfamiliar areas.
2. Turn to gum when you need extra help tackling a demanding work, school, home or creative project.
3. Pop gum in your mouth before a high-pressure event, such as a job interview (and, of course, take it out before it starts).
4. Add a pack of gum to your pens, sticky notes and other office or home essentials so it's there when you need it as you're doing day-to-day tasks.
5. Stash a stick of gum in your pocket, purse or backpack before you head out into the world in case you come across a sudden stressor or need a mood lift.
6. Stick a piece of gum in your mouth if you're experiencing anxiety while in a public place.
7. Use gum to help focus on details, for example, while tackling a spreadsheet, trying a new recipe or learning a knitting stitch.

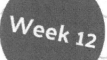

Happiness Upgrade Journal

Give yourself a Happiness Upgrade, then note where you rank on a happiness scale of 1 to 10 before and after.

Date _____

Happiness Upgrades   before   after

_____ ◯ ◯

_____ ◯ ◯

_____ ◯ ◯

Date _____

Happiness Upgrades   before   after

_____ ◯ ◯

_____ ◯ ◯

_____ ◯ ◯

Date _____

Happiness Upgrades   before   after

_____ ◯ ◯

_____ ◯ ◯

_____ ◯ ◯

Date _____

Happiness Upgrades   before   after

_____ ◯ ◯

_____ ◯ ◯

_____ ◯ ◯

Date _____

Happiness Upgrades   before   after

_____ ◯ ◯

_____ ◯ ◯

_____ ◯ ◯

Date _____

Happiness Upgrades   before   after

_____ ◯ ◯

_____ ◯ ◯

_____ ◯ ◯

Date _____

Happiness Upgrades   before   after

_____ ◯ ◯

_____ ◯ ◯

_____ ◯ ◯

Default Happiness Level

Happiness Upgrade:
Distract Yourself After a Goof

Tend to be hard on yourself when you make a mistake in front of people, such as getting someone's name wrong? Do you feel uncomfortable at parties, churning over things you said or did?

When you're in a tense social situation like this, there's an easy way to give yourself a **Happiness Upgrade**: As soon as you're able, head off somewhere and distract yourself with an activity that absorbs your whole attention. The memory of any embarrassment will fade faster and you'll be less bothered by it over the days that follow, according to research out of Wilfrid Laurier University in Canada.[1]

Why it works

Distracting your thoughts immediately after a stressful social experience interrupts the process that makes the memory permanent, helping you let it go.

Happiness Upgrade suggestions:

1. Distract yourself by playing a video game, such as Tetris.
2. Shop online or head to a store for something you need, such as office supplies, groceries or an umbrella.
3. Create something that requires intense focus, for example, bake cookies or hammer in another piece to a bookshelf you're building.
4. Grab an instrument and play a favorite tune.
5. Read a book that captures your attention, such as an exciting thriller or inspiring autobiography.
6. Rearrange part of a room or reorganize a shelf.
7. Get laughing by visiting a funny website, reading a funny book, watching a funny video or thinking back to a funny incident that puts you in stitches whenever you recall it.

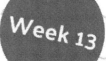

Happiness Upgrade Journal

Give yourself a Happiness Upgrade, then note where you rank on a happiness scale of 1 to 10 before and after.

Date _____

Happiness Upgrades   before   after

_____ ◯ ◯
_____ ◯ ◯
_____ ◯ ◯

Date _____

Happiness Upgrades   before   after

_____ ◯ ◯
_____ ◯ ◯
_____ ◯ ◯

Date _____

Happiness Upgrades   before   after

_____ ◯ ◯
_____ ◯ ◯
_____ ◯ ◯

Date _____

Happiness Upgrades   before   after

_____ ◯ ◯
_____ ◯ ◯
_____ ◯ ◯

Date _____

Happiness Upgrades   before   after

_____ ◯ ◯
_____ ◯ ◯
_____ ◯ ◯

Date _____

Happiness Upgrades   before   after

_____ ◯ ◯
_____ ◯ ◯
_____ ◯ ◯

Date _____

Happiness Upgrades   before   after

_____ ◯ ◯
_____ ◯ ◯
_____ ◯ ◯

Default Happiness Level

Happiness Upgrade:
Play With Your Pet

Here's a **Happiness Upgrade** built for two: Spending quality time with your cat, dog, hamster, horse or other beloved animal companion is a mood-lifter for both of you.[1] What's more, research shows that the company of pets can be even more comforting for you in times of stress than a human friend or partner.[2]

Why it works

Bonding with your pet increases the brain's production of serotonin and oxytocin, which are hormones that increase joy and calm. At the same time, it curbs the output of the stress hormone cortisol, further relaxing you.[3]

No pet around? Playing with someone else's animal pal is just as joy-boosting. In fact, it's so effective that many hospitals bring in therapy pets to visit patients as a way to raise their spirits.[3]

Happiness Upgrade suggestions:

1. Gently cuddle, stroke or kiss your cutie.
2. Grab your pet's favorite toy and get playing.
3. Get exercise for both of you by taking a walk, doing paired pet yoga or moving another way.
4. Bring a new toy to your animal pal.
5. Try to teach your bud a new trick.
6. Volunteer at shelters that rescue or rehabilitate domestic pets or wildlife.
7. Visit a cat café, dog park or other spot where there are furry friends roaming around asking to be adored.

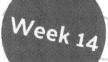

Happiness Upgrade Journal

*Give yourself a Happiness Upgrade, then note where you rank
on a happiness scale of 1 to 10 before and after.*

Date _____

Happiness Upgrades   before   after

_____   ◯ ◯

_____   ◯ ◯

_____   ◯ ◯

Date _____

Happiness Upgrades   before   after

_____   ◯ ◯

_____   ◯ ◯

_____   ◯ ◯

Date _____

Happiness Upgrades   before   after

_____   ◯ ◯

_____   ◯ ◯

_____   ◯ ◯

Date _____

Happiness Upgrades   before   after

_____   ◯ ◯

_____   ◯ ◯

_____   ◯ ◯

Date _____

Happiness Upgrades   before   after

_____   ◯ ◯

_____   ◯ ◯

_____   ◯ ◯

Date _____

Happiness Upgrades   before   after

_____   ◯ ◯

_____   ◯ ◯

_____   ◯ ◯

Date _____

Happiness Upgrades   before   after

_____   ◯ ◯

_____   ◯ ◯

_____   ◯ ◯

Default
Happiness Level

Happiness Upgrade:
Don't Put Up With Pain

If you've got a headache, backache or other discomfort, don't simply put up with it until it goes away on its own. And, don't rely on a remedy that isn't working just because it's what you've always turned to. Trying a variety of traditional and/or complementary treatments not only can bring you relief, it can also give you a **Happiness Upgrade**.

Why it works

Pain triggers changes in the body that drag down your mood, energy and brain skills.[1] Easing the ache, even a little, reverses this downward trajectory, helping you feel uplifted.

Want another reason to experiment with new ways to reduce discomfort? Research shows that a negative mood worsens pain while improving your mood lessens it.[2]

Happiness Upgrade suggestions:

1. Use over-the-counter remedies, for example, allergy medicine, antacids or painkillers.
2. Try pill-free treatments, such as a heat patch or ice pack.
3. Ask an expert about natural, safe alternative solutions, which may include caffeine, supplements or herbs.
4. Research your issue on trusted health websites (such as MayoClinic.org) to find out about other remedies.
5. Join a support group for your health issue to get recommendations from others with a similar challenge.
6. Reduce stress, a key factor that worsens pain, with meditation, progressive muscle relaxation, soft music, tai chi or another favorite relaxation method.
7. Ask your doctor, nurse, physical therapist, registered dietitian, cognitive behavioral therapist, massage therapist, pharmacist and other healthcare providers for their tips.

Happiness Upgrade Journal

*Give yourself a Happiness Upgrade, then note where you rank
on a happiness scale of 1 to 10 before and after.*

Date _____
Happiness Upgrades   before   after
_____ ◯ ◯
_____ ◯ ◯
_____ ◯ ◯

Date _____
Happiness Upgrades   before   after
_____ ◯ ◯
_____ ◯ ◯
_____ ◯ ◯

Date _____
Happiness Upgrades   before   after
_____ ◯ ◯
_____ ◯ ◯
_____ ◯ ◯

Date _____
Happiness Upgrades   before   after
_____ ◯ ◯
_____ ◯ ◯
_____ ◯ ◯

Date _____
Happiness Upgrades   before   after
_____ ◯ ◯
_____ ◯ ◯
_____ ◯ ◯

Date _____
Happiness Upgrades   before   after
_____ ◯ ◯
_____ ◯ ◯
_____ ◯ ◯

Date _____
Happiness Upgrades   before   after
_____ ◯ ◯
_____ ◯ ◯
_____ ◯ ◯

Default Happiness Level

Happiness Upgrade:
Drink a Mood Booster

Getting a **Happiness Upgrade** can be as easy as drinking a healthy, non-alcoholic beverage, such as 100% fruit juice, caffeinated tea or coffee, dark cocoa, decaffeinated coffee or tea, herbal tea, plain water, seltzer water or a spritzer made of seltzer water and 100% juice.

Why it works

Studies show that fruits, berries, dark chocolate, coffee and tea contain natural compounds, such as flavonoids, that send more nutrient-rich blood to the brain, refueling energy and positivity.[1] In moderate intakes, caffeine is a mild central nervous system stimulant that triggers the release of pep-pumping adrenaline and spurs a greater production of mood-regulating serotonin and rewarding dopamine in the brain.[2] And, drinking water or any hydrating beverage reverses mild dehydration—a common problem that causes fogginess and the blues—helping you perk up physically and emotionally.[3]

Happiness Upgrade suggestions:

1. Start your day with a refreshing glass of water.
2. Brew your favorite caffeinated drink or herbal tea.
3. Enjoy a mug of dark cocoa.
4. Pour yourself a glass of juice made from oranges, blueberries, blackberries, purple grapes or blackcurrants.
5. Mix up chocolate milk made with dark chocolate syrup.
6. Drink a fizzy glass of seltzer water straight-up or add 100% fruit juice, a squeeze of lemon, peppermint leaf, cucumber slices or another natural flavoring.
7. Try a beverage that's special or new.

Happiness Upgrade Journal

*Give yourself a Happiness Upgrade, then note where you rank
on a happiness scale of 1 to 10 before and after.*

Date _____

Happiness Upgrades   before   after

_____
_____
_____

Date _____

Happiness Upgrades   before   after

_____
_____
_____

Date _____

Happiness Upgrades   before   after

_____
_____
_____

Date _____

Happiness Upgrades   before   after

_____
_____
_____

Date _____

Happiness Upgrades   before   after

_____
_____
_____

Date _____

Happiness Upgrades   before   after

_____
_____
_____

Date _____

Happiness Upgrades   before   after

_____
_____
_____

Default
Happiness Level

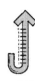

Happiness Upgrade:
Plan a Vacation

Whether you just came back from a vacation or haven't been on one in years, planning a trip you'd like to take in the future is a surefire way to get a **Happiness Upgrade** right now. Even if you don't know when you'll be able to get away, daydreaming about the sights you'd like to see and activities you'd like to do charges up your mood.

Why it works

Anticipating the fun of a vacation is exciting, which revs good feelings, reports the journal *Applied Research in Quality of Life* [1]

Can't travel far or long? Planning a short "staycation", where you enjoy activities near your home, lifts your spirits, too. That's because trips to a local museum, pick-your-own farm, amusement park and other attractions give you the sense of being away while also distracting you from your day-to-day life, according to research from Australia's University of Queensland. [2]

Happiness Upgrade suggestions:

1. Research destinations you'd like to visit on YouTube or travel websites.
2. Ask friends and family for their trip suggestions.
3. Look at photos of past vacations to get ideas for another.
4. Take steps to prepare for a trip, for example, renew your passport or get luggage.
5. Write a list of activities you've wanted to try while on vacation.
6. Think of trips you'd like to go on alone, for example, a mountain retreat or therapeutic spa.
7. Organize a group getaway with friends or family members so you can have fun planning it together.

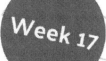

Happiness Upgrade Journal

*Give yourself a Happiness Upgrade, then note where you rank
on a happiness scale of 1 to 10 before and after.*

Date _____

Happiness Upgrades   before   after

_____   ◯ ◯
_____   ◯ ◯
_____   ◯ ◯

Date _____

Happiness Upgrades   before   after

_____   ◯ ◯
_____   ◯ ◯
_____   ◯ ◯

Date _____

Happiness Upgrades   before   after

_____   ◯ ◯
_____   ◯ ◯
_____   ◯ ◯

Date _____

Happiness Upgrades   before   after

_____   ◯ ◯
_____   ◯ ◯
_____   ◯ ◯

Date _____

Happiness Upgrades   before   after

_____   ◯ ◯
_____   ◯ ◯
_____   ◯ ◯

Date _____

Happiness Upgrades   before   after

_____   ◯ ◯
_____   ◯ ◯
_____   ◯ ◯

Date _____

Happiness Upgrades   before   after

_____   ◯ ◯
_____   ◯ ◯
_____   ◯ ◯

Default
Happiness Level

Happiness Upgrade:
Overcome Shyness With a Good Deed

Do you dread parties, networking events and other social functions because you're shy or socially anxious? If so, this can mean missing out on opportunities to make new friends, build your business, create a support network or reap other benefits that come with these kinds of activities.

Fortunately, researchers from the University of British Columbia in Canada found a way to give yourself a **Happiness Upgrade** that makes you more comfortable in social situations despite your usual unease: Do something kind for the hosts or guests.[1]

Why it works

A key cause of social anxiety is anticipating rejection or embarrassment in front of other people. Doing acts of kindness makes you anticipate a friendlier response from folks so you're more confident coming out of your shell.

Happiness Upgrade suggestions:

1. Bring food or beverages to share, such as cake, crudités or sparkling cider.
2. Ask the event organizer if there's a job you can do to help, such as hand out beverages or name tags.
3. Volunteer to assist in the event's planning.
4. Gift the host with flowers, a holiday-themed ornament or other décor in keeping with the event.
5. Compliment the hosts on the work they did for the event, such as the decorations and baking.
6. Offer to take photos and share them with the attendees.
7. Let the event coordinators know you can help clean up.

Happiness Upgrade Journal

*Give yourself a Happiness Upgrade, then note where you rank
on a happiness scale of 1 to 10 before and after.*

Date _____

Happiness Upgrades   before   after

_____   ◯ ◯
_____   ◯ ◯
_____   ◯ ◯

Date _____

Happiness Upgrades   before   after

_____   ◯ ◯
_____   ◯ ◯
_____   ◯ ◯

Date _____

Happiness Upgrades   before   after

_____   ◯ ◯
_____   ◯ ◯
_____   ◯ ◯

Date _____

Happiness Upgrades   before   after

_____   ◯ ◯
_____   ◯ ◯
_____   ◯ ◯

Date _____

Happiness Upgrades   before   after

_____   ◯ ◯
_____   ◯ ◯
_____   ◯ ◯

Date _____

Happiness Upgrades   before   after

_____   ◯ ◯
_____   ◯ ◯
_____   ◯ ◯

Date _____

Happiness Upgrades   before   after

_____   ◯ ◯
_____   ◯ ◯
_____   ◯ ◯

Default
Happiness Level

Happiness Upgrade:
Enjoy Something You Love a New Way

Have favorites you regularly turn to for a mood boost, for example, a certain meal you eat again and again or movie you've watched a hundred times? While these are great on their own, research in the journal *Personality and Social Psychology Bulletin* reveals a simple way to give them all a **Happiness Upgrade** so they're even more joy-lifting: Consume, use or experience them in a new or unusual way.[1]

Why it works

Doing activities, eating food, drinking beverages or using products in different ways than you normally do makes it feel like you're experiencing them for the first time all over again. This gives you a fresh perspective, helping you focus on what you enjoy about them.

Happiness Upgrade suggestions:

1. Eat food in a way that's different for you, such as munching popcorn with chopsticks or taking your dinner outdoors.
2. Sip beverages from unusual vessels, for example, pour orange juice into a martini glass.
3. Wear clothing, accessories or jewelry in new ways: Add a decorative pin to a hat or cuff your pants, for example.
4. Watch a movie you love someplace new, say, on a streaming device in your backyard.
5. Move a favorite chair, couch, desk or other piece of furniture into a different room of your home or set it on the porch.
6. Put photos in nontraditional frames, for example, attach them to driftwood or hold them up with pant hangers.
7. Place plants in unconventional, plant-safe pots, such as a spaghetti colander or discarded bathroom sink.

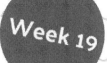

Happiness Upgrade *Journal*

*Give yourself a Happiness Upgrade, then note where you rank
on a happiness scale of 1 to 10 before and after.*

Date
Happiness Upgrades   before   after

Date
Happiness Upgrades   before   after

Date
Happiness Upgrades   before   after

Date
Happiness Upgrades   before   after

Date
Happiness Upgrades   before   after

Date
Happiness Upgrades   before   after

Date
Happiness Upgrades   before   after

Default
Happiness Level

Happiness Upgrade:
Sing

Whether you need to reverse a sagging mood or want to intensify the joy that you're currently feeling, you can give yourself a **Happiness Upgrade** by belting out a song. Regardless of whether you hit the right notes or sing the correct lyrics, the simple act of singing is a proven way to elevate positivity fast.

Why it works

Singing spurs your body's production of endocannabinoids, which are molecules that cause a euphoric sensation similar to a "runner's high" where mood, confidence and relaxation all peak.[1] Crooning a tune also decreases the stress hormone cortisol, helping to usher in greater calm.[2]

Happiness Upgrade suggestions:

1. Create a playlist of songs you love, then sing along to them when you want a quick mood boost.
2. Keep a list of songs you like to sing *a cappella* (without music) nearby, such as in a desk drawer, so you can instantly pick one.
3. Wake up to an alarm that plays favorite songs or keep a music device near your bed and turn it on after awakening.
4. Try out acoustics in different areas to find more fun places to sing, such as your shower (naturally) or car (the dashboard resonates your voice).
5. Compile songs to match tasks during the day, for instance, fast tempo songs to help you plow through physically intensive to-dos and slow tempo songs when relaxing.
6. Find new songs to sing by asking friends what they love.
7. Take a trip down memory lane and sing songs that made you happy when you were younger.

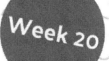

Week 20

Happiness Upgrade Journal

Give yourself a Happiness Upgrade, then note where you rank on a happiness scale of 1 to 10 before and after.

Date _____
Happiness Upgrades   before   after
_____   ○   ○
_____   ○   ○
_____   ○   ○

Date _____
Happiness Upgrades   before   after
_____   ○   ○
_____   ○   ○
_____   ○   ○

Date _____
Happiness Upgrades   before   after
_____   ○   ○
_____   ○   ○
_____   ○   ○

Date _____
Happiness Upgrades   before   after
_____   ○   ○
_____   ○   ○
_____   ○   ○

Date _____
Happiness Upgrades   before   after
_____   ○   ○
_____   ○   ○
_____   ○   ○

Date _____
Happiness Upgrades   before   after
_____   ○   ○
_____   ○   ○
_____   ○   ○

Date _____
Happiness Upgrades   before   after
_____   ○   ○
_____   ○   ○
_____   ○   ○

Default
Happiness Level

Happiness Upgrade:
Smell Fragrant Flowers

You may have heard the old adage "Stop and smell the roses", which means that pausing to enjoy life's little pleasures can make you happier. Well, research shows that you'll give yourself a **Happiness Upgrade** when you *literally* stop and smell roses as well as any other fragrant flower, such as gardenias, honeysuckle, hyacinths, lavender, lilacs and jasmine.[1]

Why it works

When you inhale the scent of fragrant blooms, compounds that give them their unique scents, such as linalool, get absorbed into nasal membranes, then travel to the brain. Once there, these odor molecules have beneficial effects on areas that impact mood and stress.

Happiness Upgrade suggestions:

1. Place a potted flowering scented plant where you spend a lot of your time, such as your desk or a nearby counter.
2. Fill a vase with scented flowers and put it in an area where you can easily take sniffs of them throughout the day.
3. Stash a vase with fragrant blooms someplace surprising that you visit at least once a day, such as the bathroom.
4. Dab on an essential oil of your favorite flowery fragrance or add a few drops to a cotton ball and sniff.
5. Keep a bowl of naturally-scented floral potpourri by your bedside (far from curious pets and children) so it's the first aroma you inhale when starting your day and the last aroma you inhale before falling asleep.
6. Pause in stores that sell aromatic flowers, such as your local food market, to get a whiff.
7. Take a "flower walk" around your neighborhood or in a park and pause to inhale as many floral aromas as you can find.

Happiness Upgrade Journal

Give yourself a Happiness Upgrade, then note where you rank on a happiness scale of 1 to 10 before and after.

Date _____

Happiness Upgrades   before   after
_____ ○ ○
_____ ○ ○
_____ ○ ○

Date _____

Happiness Upgrades   before   after
_____ ○ ○
_____ ○ ○
_____ ○ ○

Date _____

Happiness Upgrades   before   after
_____ ○ ○
_____ ○ ○
_____ ○ ○

Date _____

Happiness Upgrades   before   after
_____ ○ ○
_____ ○ ○
_____ ○ ○

Date _____

Happiness Upgrades   before   after
_____ ○ ○
_____ ○ ○
_____ ○ ○

Date _____

Happiness Upgrades   before   after
_____ ○ ○
_____ ○ ○
_____ ○ ○

Date _____

Happiness Upgrades   before   after
_____ ○ ○
_____ ○ ○
_____ ○ ○

Default Happiness Level

Happiness Upgrade:
Enjoy a Fun Break

While in the middle of a task, do you put off enjoying a bit of fun, such as chatting with a friend, because you think you'll feel guilty when there's still work left to do? If so, you'll get a **Happiness Upgrade** by granting yourself permission to take a short fun break before you're finished. Researchers from the University of Chicago found that taking a pleasurable time-out from a task, then resuming it afterward, boosts your mood immediately *without* regret.[1] Indeed, in their study, volunteers who took a fun break while in the middle of a project felt no remorse and were happier for doing it.

Why it works

According to the study authors, many of us tend to overestimate how irresponsible we'll feel if we put fun ahead of work. As a result, we may continually postpone favorite activities until the time is right. But, turns out, our worry is unfounded. Even if you're in the middle of a task, it doesn't reduce the pleasure you get from doing something you love. In fact, an entertaining time-out can rejuvenate you, making you even more focused and productive once you return to your to-dos.

Happiness Upgrade suggestions:

1. Read a few pages or one chapter in a book.
2. Play a musical instrument you enjoy.
3. Add to an art project, such a collage, painting or scrapbook.
4. Enjoy a leisurely walk or stimulating workout.
5. Pamper yourself, for example, with self-massage.
6. Call a friend or family member to chat.
7. Hop in your car, on your bike or on a bus for a mini exploration.

Happiness Upgrade Journal

*Give yourself a Happiness Upgrade, then note where you rank
on a happiness scale of 1 to 10 before and after.*

Date _____
Happiness Upgrades   before   after
_____   ◯ ◯
_____   ◯ ◯
_____   ◯ ◯

Date _____
Happiness Upgrades   before   after
_____   ◯ ◯
_____   ◯ ◯
_____   ◯ ◯

Date _____
Happiness Upgrades   before   after
_____   ◯ ◯
_____   ◯ ◯
_____   ◯ ◯

Date _____
Happiness Upgrades   before   after
_____   ◯ ◯
_____   ◯ ◯
_____   ◯ ◯

Date _____
Happiness Upgrades   before   after
_____   ◯ ◯
_____   ◯ ◯
_____   ◯ ◯

Date _____
Happiness Upgrades   before   after
_____   ◯ ◯
_____   ◯ ◯
_____   ◯ ◯

Date _____
Happiness Upgrades   before   after
_____   ◯ ◯
_____   ◯ ◯
_____   ◯ ◯

Default
Happiness Level

Happiness Upgrade:
Opt for Good Enough

Ever feel paralyzed when trying to make a choice, for example, what to buy or do, because you keep weighing the pros and cons to ensure you make the *very best choice*? Instead of stressing yourself out and delaying your decision, give yourself a **Happiness Upgrade** by settling on an option that's *good enough*. Research shows that folks who follow this advice are more satisfied with their decisions and happier overall.[1]

Why it works

Striving for the perfect choice is mentally exhausting, gobbles up your time, prolongs your anxiety and sets you up for regret when you find yet another "perfect" option after you've chosen. Deciding to settle on a selection that fulfills most of your key needs without being perfect gives you instant relief, allowing you to relax and move on.

Happiness Upgrade suggestions:

1. When faced with a large number of options for a big decision, such as which of 10 different laptops to buy, limit your research to three trusted sources (such as websites or podcasts), then follow the experts' advice.
2. Go with what your gut tells you is right.
3. When it seems like all the choices are equal, make your pick at random just for fun.
4. Have a person in charge make a recommendation, for example, ask a barista at a café when choosing coffee or librarian when borrowing a book.
5. Ask a friend or family member what they would choose.
6. Give yourself a deadline to make your choice, for example, 24 hours to decide which event to attend.
7. Go with what you've already had in the past.

Happiness Upgrade Journal

*Give yourself a Happiness Upgrade, then note where you rank
on a happiness scale of 1 to 10 before and after.*

Date _____

Happiness Upgrades   before   after

_____   ○   ○
_____   ○   ○
_____   ○   ○

Date _____

Happiness Upgrades   before   after

_____   ○   ○
_____   ○   ○
_____   ○   ○

Date _____

Happiness Upgrades   before   after

_____   ○   ○
_____   ○   ○
_____   ○   ○

Date _____

Happiness Upgrades   before   after

_____   ○   ○
_____   ○   ○
_____   ○   ○

Date _____

Happiness Upgrades   before   after

_____   ○   ○
_____   ○   ○
_____   ○   ○

Date _____

Happiness Upgrades   before   after

_____   ○   ○
_____   ○   ○
_____   ○   ○

Date _____

Happiness Upgrades   before   after

_____   ○   ○
_____   ○   ○
_____   ○   ○

Default Happiness Level

Happiness Upgrade:
Seek Out a Smile

As simple as it seems, you can give yourself a **Happiness Upgrade** by just looking other people's joyous smiles.

Why it works

Seeing someone else's happy face activates specific regions in the brain (such as the hippocampus, amygdala and parahippocampal gyrus) that make you happy, too, according to an fMRI study out of Germany's University of Tübingen.[1] Researchers theorize that humans may be naturally wired to match the emotion of another person they see as a way to improve communication.

Happiness Upgrade suggestions:

1. Head to a nearby park where folks are enjoying a beautiful day.
2. Visit a dog run where pooches and their pet parents are running around and throwing balls.
3. Seek out places where folks are happy to be taking a break from their everyday lives, for example, head to a tourist destination, such as a beach. Or, visit a popular entertainment destination for locals, such as a skating rink.
4. Sneak peeks inside a bakery where customers are looking forward to indulging in sweet temptations.
5. Enjoy a live comedy or improv show where there are smiles and laughs aplenty.
6. Cue up a video on YouTube of someone who's known for their bubbly, ever-smiling personality.
7. During festive holidays, make a beeline to displays and activities where people gather to enjoy the special occasion.

Happiness Upgrade Journal

*Give yourself a Happiness Upgrade, then note where you rank
on a happiness scale of 1 to 10 before and after.*

Date _____
Happiness Upgrades   before   after
_____   ○ ○
_____   ○ ○
_____   ○ ○

Date _____
Happiness Upgrades   before   after
_____   ○ ○
_____   ○ ○
_____   ○ ○

Date _____
Happiness Upgrades   before   after
_____   ○ ○
_____   ○ ○
_____   ○ ○

Date _____
Happiness Upgrades   before   after
_____   ○ ○
_____   ○ ○
_____   ○ ○

Date _____
Happiness Upgrades   before   after
_____   ○ ○
_____   ○ ○
_____   ○ ○

Date _____
Happiness Upgrades   before   after
_____   ○ ○
_____   ○ ○
_____   ○ ○

Date _____
Happiness Upgrades   before   after
_____   ○ ○
_____   ○ ○
_____   ○ ○

Default
Happiness Level

Happiness Upgrade:
Take a Risk

When you're hankering for a quick **Happiness Upgrade**, consider taking a safe, but thrilling risk. Folks who take a chance on something not only get an instant surge of good feelings, they're happier with their lives than those who never take a leap of faith, research shows.[1] And, this holds true regardless of the outcome.

Why it works

Taking a risk immediately prompts the body to churn out pleasure-inducing chemicals, such as dopamine and adrenaline.[2] Plus, despite the uncertain outcome, risk-taking makes you feel like you're more in control of your life by giving you an opportunity to go after something you want, which researchers have found is tied closely to happiness levels.[3]

Happiness Upgrade suggestions:

1. Dare to step outside your comfort zone, for example, by singing at an open mic event or filming yourself dancing in public for a fun social media challenge.
2. Ask someone new out on a romantic date or ask someone new out on a platonic friend date.
3. Try a new look, for instance, wear a different type of outfit than you usually do or style your hair differently.
4. Enter a competition, for example, submit one of your photos, recipes or songs.
5. Send in your application to a dream job or ask for a raise or promotion at your current job.
6. Throw a dart at a map of your local area, then visit wherever it lands.
7. Strike up a conversation with a stranger.

Happiness Upgrade *Journal*

Give yourself a Happiness Upgrade, then note where you rank on a happiness scale of 1 to 10 before and after.

Date _____

Happiness Upgrades before after

_____ ◯ ◯
_____ ◯ ◯
_____ ◯ ◯

Date _____

Happiness Upgrades before after

_____ ◯ ◯
_____ ◯ ◯
_____ ◯ ◯

Date _____

Happiness Upgrades before after

_____ ◯ ◯
_____ ◯ ◯
_____ ◯ ◯

Date _____

Happiness Upgrades before after

_____ ◯ ◯
_____ ◯ ◯
_____ ◯ ◯

Date _____

Happiness Upgrades before after

_____ ◯ ◯
_____ ◯ ◯
_____ ◯ ◯

Date _____

Happiness Upgrades before after

_____ ◯ ◯
_____ ◯ ◯
_____ ◯ ◯

Date _____

Happiness Upgrades before after

_____ ◯ ◯
_____ ◯ ◯
_____ ◯ ◯

Default
Happiness Level

Happiness Upgrade:
Carry a Lucky Charm

Do you believe certain objects have the power to boost your luck, for example, a coin you found on the ground? Think a certain gesture you make can improve outcomes, such as crossing your fingers? If so, you can give yourself a **Happiness Upgrade** by carrying the lucky charm with you or performing the gesture whenever you need an extra dose of luck. Research shows that folks who put faith in lucky objects or rituals are more optimistic, hopeful and confident.[1]

Why it works

Believing in the power of luck-boosters makes you feel like you have an added advantage, which increases your confidence that you'll do better. In turn, you actually do perform better at whatever task you take on. Indeed, in multiple studies, folks relying on lucky charms or gestures outperformed those without them.

Happiness Upgrade suggestions:

1. Designate a spot on you to keep your lucky charm, such as in a pocket, then place it there whenever you need a boost.
2. Be on the lookout for a new lucky charm, which can be anything (such as a coin or toy) that makes you confident.
3. Ask friends for recommendations on what they believe is a lucky token or gesture since it might work for you, too.
4. Find out if your family has any luck-boosting traditions.
5. Research if there are any lucky charms from your culture.
6. Craft your own original good luck charm. This could mean painting a stone, carving wood or decoupaging an object.
7. Infuse a lucky charm with more power by asking someone you feel is particularly lucky to hold it for a moment.

Happiness Upgrade Journal

*Give yourself a Happiness Upgrade, then note where you rank
on a happiness scale of 1 to 10 before and after.*

Date _____
Happiness Upgrades before after

Date _____
Happiness Upgrades before after

Date _____
Happiness Upgrades before after

Date _____
Happiness Upgrades before after

Date _____
Happiness Upgrades before after

Date _____
Happiness Upgrades before after

Date _____
Happiness Upgrades before after

Default
Happiness Level

Happiness Upgrade:
Get Moving

No doubt you've heard that one of the most important ways to improve your health is by exercising. Well, good news, working out at any intensity—low, medium or high—for at least 15 minutes also gives you a mood-boosting **Happiness Upgrade** that starts immediately and lasts up to 24 hours.[1] And, this joy-lifting benefit kicks in whether you're new to working out or an avid exerciser.

Why it works

Exercise triggers the production of certain chemicals that elevate emotions, such as dopamine, endorphins, norepinephrine and serotonin. What's more, working out improves body image and self-esteem after a single session, regardless of body shape, by making you feel stronger and fitter.[2]

Happiness Upgrade suggestions:

1. Head outdoors for a bike ride, hike, jog, skate, swim or walk.
2. When indoors, hop on a treadmill, stationary bike or other favorite type of gym equipment.
3. Climb up and down stairs.
4. Do exercises in place, such as jumping jacks, push-ups or squats.
5. Strengthen your muscles with isometric exercises, resistance bands or weights.
6. Join a live in-person or virtual exercise class, such as cardio, cycling or kickboxing or follow along to a pre-recorded video.
7. Make moving fun, for example, pick up a hula hoop, play badminton or dance.

Happiness Upgrade Journal

*Give yourself a Happiness Upgrade, then note where you rank
on a happiness scale of 1 to 10 before and after.*

Date _____

Happiness Upgrades   before   after

_____   ◯   ◯
_____   ◯   ◯
_____   ◯   ◯
_____

Date _____

Happiness Upgrades   before   after

_____   ◯   ◯
_____   ◯   ◯
_____   ◯   ◯
_____

Date _____

Happiness Upgrades   before   after

_____   ◯   ◯
_____   ◯   ◯
_____   ◯   ◯
_____

Date _____

Happiness Upgrades   before   after

_____   ◯   ◯
_____   ◯   ◯
_____   ◯   ◯
_____

Date _____

Happiness Upgrades   before   after

_____   ◯   ◯
_____   ◯   ◯
_____   ◯   ◯
_____

Date _____

Happiness Upgrades   before   after

_____   ◯   ◯
_____   ◯   ◯
_____   ◯   ◯
_____

Date _____

Happiness Upgrades   before   after

_____   ◯   ◯
_____   ◯   ◯
_____   ◯   ◯
_____

**Default
Happiness Level**

Happiness Upgrade:
Change the Subject

Ever find your mood going down when chatting with someone who's in a bad mood? You could be "catching" their grumpiness. Researchers found that, like a cold, negative emotions are contagious, spreading from one person to the next.[1] If you can't walk away from the person (for instance, because they're a loved one or client), there is a way you can give yourself a **Happiness Upgrade** when in their company: Switch the conversation topic to one that's uplifting. You'll both feel lighter within minutes.

Why it works

When you're in the company of someone who's in a bad mood, you tend to automatically mimic their negative body language and facial expressions, such as a furrowed brow, hunched shoulders or frown. These physical cues then tell your brain that this is an emotion *you're* feeling so it churns out chemicals to match it, spurring the same unhappy emotion in you. Luckily, good moods are just as contagious. So, when you inspire happiness in someone else, it lifts you up, too.

Happiness Upgrade suggestions:

1. Ask the person to recall a positive moment in their day.
2. Pivot the conversation away from stressful topics to one that's joyful, for example, share good news you heard.
3. Point out something beautiful going on near where you're talking, such as a flowering plant.
4. Help the person see a silver lining.
5. Make a light-hearted joke the other person would find funny.
6. Ask the person to imagine a scenario where an issue they're facing is resolved positively and to describe it.
7. Be transparent and tell the person you'd like to change the topic to one that's more uplifting.

Happiness Upgrade Journal

*Give yourself a Happiness Upgrade, then note where you rank
on a happiness scale of 1 to 10 before and after.*

Date _____

Happiness Upgrades   before   after

_____   ◯   ◯
_____   ◯   ◯
_____   ◯   ◯

Date _____

Happiness Upgrades   before   after

_____   ◯   ◯
_____   ◯   ◯
_____   ◯   ◯

Date _____

Happiness Upgrades   before   after

_____   ◯   ◯
_____   ◯   ◯
_____   ◯   ◯

Date _____

Happiness Upgrades   before   after

_____   ◯   ◯
_____   ◯   ◯
_____   ◯   ◯

Date _____

Happiness Upgrades   before   after

_____   ◯   ◯
_____   ◯   ◯
_____   ◯   ◯

Date _____

Happiness Upgrades   before   after

_____   ◯   ◯
_____   ◯   ◯
_____   ◯   ◯

Date _____

Happiness Upgrades   before   after

_____   ◯   ◯
_____   ◯   ◯
_____   ◯   ◯

Default
Happiness Level

Happiness Upgrade:
Cut Yourself Some Slack

You know those warm words of comfort that you say to friends and family who need a lift when things go wrong in their life? You can give yourself a **Happiness Upgrade** by showing yourself the same compassion that you give to them. Research shows that comforting yourself as you would a loved one when you slip up or don't meet your expectations leads to greater inner peace in the moment and higher satisfaction with your life, in general.[1]

Why it works

Fostering self-compassion makes it easier for you to embrace your own flaws and limitations, which reduces stress. If you're a perfectionist, self-compassion also helps you cope when you don't live up to the high ideals you often strive to meet. As a result, you're less critical and more accepting of yourself.

Happiness Upgrade suggestions:

1. Create a phrase to say when you're being hard on yourself, such as, "I'm doing my best, which is enough."
2. Think about a pep talk that you'd say to someone you love if they didn't reach a goal, then give yourself the same talk.
3. Reward yourself when you show self-compassion, for example, treating yourself to a fresh cup of tea.
4. Set lower, more realistic expectations for yourself.
5. For non-essential tasks (such as cleaning a room), tell yourself, "It doesn't have to be perfect. It just has to be done."
6. Recall instances when you did well in the past so you can feel proud of former achievements.
7. Forgive yourself for any shortcomings, reminding yourself that there's always room for growth for everyone.

Happiness Upgrade Journal

*Give yourself a Happiness Upgrade, then note where you rank
on a happiness scale of 1 to 10 before and after.*

Date _____
Happiness Upgrades before after
_____
_____
_____

Date _____
Happiness Upgrades before after
_____
_____
_____

Date _____
Happiness Upgrades before after
_____
_____
_____

Date _____
Happiness Upgrades before after
_____
_____
_____

Date _____
Happiness Upgrades before after
_____
_____
_____

Date _____
Happiness Upgrades before after
_____
_____
_____

Date _____
Happiness Upgrades before after
_____
_____
_____

Default Happiness Level

Happiness Upgrade:
Give Someone a Gift

Treating yourself to a gift every once in a while is a surefire way to boost cheer. And, researchers say that giving a gift to *someone else* leads to an even bigger **Happiness Upgrade**. The proof: In multiple studies, volunteers who were asked to spend money either on themselves or others experienced greater, longer-lasting joy when splurging on another person.[1]

Why it works

Being generous to others makes you feel better about yourself because it reminds you that you're kind. Plus, it helps strengthen your bonds with others. Best of all: You don't have to spend a lot of cash—or even any money at all—to rev positivity. Any type of gift you offer to someone triggers a bump in happiness.

Happiness Upgrade suggestions:

1. Bake, cook or purchase food and bring it to a friend.
2. Give a plant you've grown to a garden lover.
3. Mail a postcard, greeting card or letter to someone thanking them for something they did for you (for example, if they were a former mentor), complimenting them on an achievement (such as graduating school) or simply letting them know you're thinking about them.
4. Send a small gift card for a coffee or meal to someone who you think could use a lift.
5. Drop thank-you cards on the cars of frontline workers, for example, at hospitals and firehouses.
6. Leave gifts for others to find on their own, for instance, paint inspiring messages or uplifting images on rocks and scatter them around town.
7. Bring a bag of groceries to your local food bank or pet food to a nearby animal shelter.

Happiness Upgrade Journal

*Give yourself a Happiness Upgrade, then note where you rank
on a happiness scale of 1 to 10 before and after.*

Date _____
Happiness Upgrades   before   after
_____ ◯ ◯
_____ ◯ ◯
_____ ◯ ◯

Date _____
Happiness Upgrades   before   after
_____ ◯ ◯
_____ ◯ ◯
_____ ◯ ◯

Date _____
Happiness Upgrades   before   after
_____ ◯ ◯
_____ ◯ ◯
_____ ◯ ◯

Date _____
Happiness Upgrades   before   after
_____ ◯ ◯
_____ ◯ ◯
_____ ◯ ◯

Date _____
Happiness Upgrades   before   after
_____ ◯ ◯
_____ ◯ ◯
_____ ◯ ◯

Date _____
Happiness Upgrades   before   after
_____ ◯ ◯
_____ ◯ ◯
_____ ◯ ◯

Date _____
Happiness Upgrades   before   after
_____ ◯ ◯
_____ ◯ ◯
_____ ◯ ◯

Default
Happiness Level

Happiness Upgrade:
Save Some for Later

Next time you're enjoying a fun activity or tucking into a favorite food, try using this easy tactic to give yourself a bigger **Happiness Upgrade**: Instead of finishing off the whole thing at once, save some for later.

Why it works

A University of Michigan study shows that our favorite part of a pleasurable experience is the last bit.[1] That's because you're aware that the experience is close to ending so you focus all your energy into savoring what's left, which heightens your sensations, attention and appreciation. This means by simply dividing up what you're doing or consuming, you get to relish the best part again and again.

Happiness Upgrade suggestions:

1. Instead of eating a full serving of a favorite food in one sitting, such as a bowl of ice cream, separate it into at least two smaller servings to enjoy at different times.
2. Pour your daily coffee, tea, juice or other beverage into a smaller cup, then give yourself a refreshing refill.
3. When reading a book for pleasure, try to hold off continuing into the next chapter (despite any cliffhanger!) until later.
4. If you want to binge-watch a TV show, consider watching just two episodes at a time rather than an entire season.
5. Schedule a break in the middle of an activity you enjoy, such as visiting a museum, swimming at the beach or playing a video game, then resume your fun.
6. Divide a longer activity, such as visiting a nature preserve or theme park, into more than one day.
7. When chatting with a friend or family member, instead of catching up all at once, plan two or more shorter chats.

Happiness Upgrade Journal

Give yourself a Happiness Upgrade, then note where you rank on a happiness scale of 1 to 10 before and after.

Date _____

Happiness Upgrades before after

_____ ○ ○
_____ ○ ○
_____ ○ ○
_____

Date _____

Happiness Upgrades before after

_____ ○ ○
_____ ○ ○
_____ ○ ○
_____

Date _____

Happiness Upgrades before after

_____ ○ ○
_____ ○ ○
_____ ○ ○
_____

Date _____

Happiness Upgrades before after

_____ ○ ○
_____ ○ ○
_____ ○ ○
_____

Date _____

Happiness Upgrades before after

_____ ○ ○
_____ ○ ○
_____ ○ ○
_____

Date _____

Happiness Upgrades before after

_____ ○ ○
_____ ○ ○
_____ ○ ○
_____

Date _____

Happiness Upgrades before after

_____ ○ ○
_____ ○ ○
_____ ○ ○
_____

Default Happiness Level

Happiness Upgrade:
Put Positive Thoughts in Your Pocket

For a customized **Happiness Upgrade** you can take with you on the go, write what you like about yourself on a piece of paper. It could be your personality traits, talents, skills, achievements, appearance or anything else you admire. Then, fold the paper and place it in your pocket or anywhere else where it's easy for you to tote around. Simply carrying around these positive thoughts makes you feel better about yourself, even if you don't look at the note again, according to a study in the journal *Psychological Science*.[1]

Why it works

Writing down uplifting statements about yourself, then carrying that piece of paper on you, makes your thoughts feel like physical possessions. As a result, they have a more powerful impact on your mood. By contrast, throwing away a note with a message on it makes those thoughts fade away, the same study found. So, if you have any negative self-views you'd like to erase from your mind, write them down, then toss them in the trash.

Happiness Upgrade suggestions:

1. Write what you like most about your personality.
2. Jot down skills you're proud to be learning or have already learned.
3. List achievements you've earned.
4. Describe your body or appearance in positive terms.
5. Remind yourself of what makes you special, such as a talent or your ability to comfort friends in need.
6. Recall a compliment someone gave you that you appreciated.
7. Give yourself a compliment.

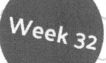

Week 32

Happiness Upgrade Journal

Give yourself a Happiness Upgrade, then note where you rank on a happiness scale of 1 to 10 before and after.

Date _____
Happiness Upgrades before after

Date _____
Happiness Upgrades before after

Date _____
Happiness Upgrades before after

Date _____
Happiness Upgrades before after

Date _____
Happiness Upgrades before after

Date _____
Happiness Upgrades before after

Date _____
Happiness Upgrades before after

Default Happiness Level

Happiness Upgrade:
Take a Stroll Anywhere

An instant **Happiness Upgrade** is as close as your own two feet, according to an Iowa State University study. In a series of three experiments, scientists discovered that walking anywhere for any length of time at any speed, even on a treadmill, is all it takes to lift your mood.[1] What's more, this joy-boosting benefit holds true regardless of weather conditions, what you see around you or what you think about while on the walk.

More surprisingly, the study also found that even if you expect walking to have a negative effect on your outlook, you'll still get a bump in positivity. This means it's worth it to get tromping even if you're convinced it's just a waste of time since you'll end up feeling at least a little more uplifted than if you stayed put.

Why it works

The study authors theorize that humans are naturally wired to get a mood boost from walking because we evolved to connect it with finding food and water. So, it may be an ancient mechanism that ties the kind of movement needed to forage with pleasant rewards.

Happiness Upgrade suggestions:

1. Start off your day on a brighter note by ambling around the block, your neighborhood or a nearby park.
2. Take stroll breaks throughout your day.
3. If you're indoors and can't go outside, saunter to the kitchen or another part of your home, workplace or building.
4. Circle the room at parties and other social events.
5. Hop on a treadmill.
6. Take a friend with you on a hike for a mutual mood boost.
7. See if you can nudge a good mood even higher with a walk.

Happiness Upgrade Journal

Give yourself a Happiness Upgrade, then note where you rank on a happiness scale of 1 to 10 before and after.

Date _____

Happiness Upgrades   before   after

_____   ◯   ◯

_____   ◯   ◯

_____   ◯   ◯

Date _____

Happiness Upgrades   before   after

_____   ◯   ◯

_____   ◯   ◯

_____   ◯   ◯

Date _____

Happiness Upgrades   before   after

_____   ◯   ◯

_____   ◯   ◯

_____   ◯   ◯

Date _____

Happiness Upgrades   before   after

_____   ◯   ◯

_____   ◯   ◯

_____   ◯   ◯

Date _____

Happiness Upgrades   before   after

_____   ◯   ◯

_____   ◯   ◯

_____   ◯   ◯

Date _____

Happiness Upgrades   before   after

_____   ◯   ◯

_____   ◯   ◯

_____   ◯   ◯

Date _____

Happiness Upgrades   before   after

_____   ◯   ◯

_____   ◯   ◯

_____   ◯   ◯

Default Happiness Level

Happiness Upgrade:
Savor a Pleasant Moment

Next time you're enjoying something pleasant, such your first sip of coffee for the day, give yourself a **Happiness Upgrade** by pausing. Ponder what makes this experience wonderful. Think about how it makes you feel. Then, see if you can prolong the enjoyment just a few seconds more. Taking time to savor positive moments raises inner joy in the moment and increases uplifting feelings throughout your day.[1]

Why it works

Savoring pleasurable experiences makes you more aware that they're happening so they have a more intense impact on you. On top of that, it trains your brain to look for additional pleasant moments in your day that you might otherwise miss, giving you even more opportunities for a mood boost.

Happiness Upgrade suggestions:

1. When you're about to do something you enjoy (for example, taking a sip of cocoa), wait a moment, then remind yourself to slow down and think about why you like it so much.
2. Upon stepping outside, pause and contemplate how transitioning to the outdoors makes you feel.
3. In the middle of a shower or bath, focus on the sensation of water on your skin or the scent of your soap.
4. When your bare feet touch a new surface (such as a fuzzy rug), think about what it feels like. Wiggle your toes.
5. As you eat, savor the taste and texture of the food.
6. During a restful break, ponder what you're doing to unplug and how it helps you reboot.
7. After lying down to sleep, pay attention to those first few moments when your body is able to relax and let go.

Happiness Upgrade Journal

*Give yourself a Happiness Upgrade, then note where you rank
on a happiness scale of 1 to 10 before and after.*

Date _____
Happiness Upgrades   before   after

Date _____
Happiness Upgrades   before   after

Date _____
Happiness Upgrades   before   after

Date _____
Happiness Upgrades   before   after

Date _____
Happiness Upgrades   before   after

Date _____
Happiness Upgrades   before   after

Date _____
Happiness Upgrades   before   after

Default
Happiness Level

Happiness Upgrade:
Gaze at Something Awe-Inspiring

One surefire way to give yourself a **Happiness Upgrade**? Look at anything that inspires awe, for example, stroll through a park with tall trees or search online for historic monuments. Whether you see them in person or on a screen, gazing at breathtaking views gives you an instant lift in positivity.[1]

Why it works

Experiencing awe pivots your thoughts away from your inner world to the vast world outside you. This helps put life in perspective and makes you feel more connected to something larger than yourself.

Happiness Upgrade suggestions:

1. Head outdoors where you can gaze at a sunrise, sunset, blue sky, fluffy clouds or twinkling nighttime stars.
2. Visit an area with awe-inspiring natural scenery, such as waterfalls, a forest or botanical gardens.
3. Stroll along the shoreline of a beach, lake or other body of water or walk along a pier.
4. Walk through a historic part of your town.
5. Head to the top of a hill or tall building and look out at the view.
6. Explore a museum in person or online.
7. Visit monuments, historical sites, cities, remote towns and natural wonders around the world virtually by using the "street view" function on Google.com/maps. Simply select your desired destination, pick up the yellow figure from the "Explore" menu, then drop it into the street map, which allows you to take 360-degree walking tours.

Happiness Upgrade Journal

*Give yourself a Happiness Upgrade, then note where you rank
on a happiness scale of 1 to 10 before and after.*

Date _____
Happiness Upgrades   before   after
_____   ◯ ◯
_____   ◯ ◯
_____   ◯ ◯

Date _____
Happiness Upgrades   before   after
_____   ◯ ◯
_____   ◯ ◯
_____   ◯ ◯

Date _____
Happiness Upgrades   before   after
_____   ◯ ◯
_____   ◯ ◯
_____   ◯ ◯

Date _____
Happiness Upgrades   before   after
_____   ◯ ◯
_____   ◯ ◯
_____   ◯ ◯

Date _____
Happiness Upgrades   before   after
_____   ◯ ◯
_____   ◯ ◯
_____   ◯ ◯

Date _____
Happiness Upgrades   before   after
_____   ◯ ◯
_____   ◯ ◯
_____   ◯ ◯

Date _____
Happiness Upgrades   before   after
_____   ◯ ◯
_____   ◯ ◯
_____   ◯ ◯

Default Happiness Level

Happiness Upgrade:
Indulge Yourself

Have trouble fully enjoying "guilty pleasures", such as watching television purely for entertainment, because you think you should be doing something more productive? Give yourself a **Happiness Upgrade** by allowing yourself to enjoy indulgent activities without any of the guilt. Research in the journal *Personality and Social Psychology Bulletin* shows that folks who follow this advice are happier in the moment, and also happier with their life, in general.[1]

Why it works

As the researchers explain it, we often believe pursuing goals that require self-control, such as working on a task or exercising, leads to greater happiness than slacking off. But, truth is, the ability to enjoy indulgent pleasures without thoughts of regret is equally important to feeling happy and satisfied with life. That's because it gives you the opportunity to relax and destress, which reboots your mind and body.

Happiness Upgrade suggestions:

1. Add an indulgent activity to your calendar to avoid guilt from taking time away from another task.
2. Enjoy your activity in a place where you can't see reminders of work, school, family, exercise or other responsibilities.
3. Silence electronic devices that ring or send you notifications before doing your activity so you can focus on it.
4. Remind yourself of the benefits of indulgent pleasures, such as a better mood and lower stress.
5. Invite a pal to enjoy an indulgent pleasure with you.
6. Use your imagination to think of new fun pleasures to try.
7. Reward yourself when you successfully enjoy an indulgent activity without guilt.

Happiness Upgrade Journal

*Give yourself a Happiness Upgrade, then note where you rank
on a happiness scale of 1 to 10 before and after.*

Date _____

Happiness Upgrades   before   after

_____ ◯ ◯

_____ ◯ ◯

_____ ◯ ◯

Date _____

Happiness Upgrades   before   after

_____ ◯ ◯

_____ ◯ ◯

_____ ◯ ◯

Date _____

Happiness Upgrades   before   after

_____ ◯ ◯

_____ ◯ ◯

_____ ◯ ◯

Date _____

Happiness Upgrades   before   after

_____ ◯ ◯

_____ ◯ ◯

_____ ◯ ◯

Date _____

Happiness Upgrades   before   after

_____ ◯ ◯

_____ ◯ ◯

_____ ◯ ◯

Date _____

Happiness Upgrades   before   after

_____ ◯ ◯

_____ ◯ ◯

_____ ◯ ◯

Date _____

Happiness Upgrades   before   after

_____ ◯ ◯

_____ ◯ ◯

_____ ◯ ◯

Default
Happiness Level

Happiness Upgrade:
Dance to Groovy Music

Try to notice the next time you're in a "flow" state, which is when you're so engrossed in an activity you love (such as creating art, gardening or exercising) that you forget about all sense of time and space. Then, give yourself a **Happiness Upgrade** by turning on music with a syncopated beat (with or without lyrics) and dance. You'll intensify your flow state, making it even more pleasurable, shows a study from Canada's International Laboratory for Brain, Music and Sound Research.[1]

Why it works

The rhythmic movement of dancing heightens your flow state by distracting you from self-critical thoughts and spurring a greater production of mood-boosting dopamine and endorphins.

Happiness Upgrade suggestions:

1. While creating art, such as a painting or sculpture, crank up danceable tunes and let the music move you.
2. Before working on your yard or garden, don headphones and call up your favorite shimmy-worthy playlist.
3. While brainstorming ideas for work, school or projects, turn on music with an invigorating beat.
4. When playing your own music on an instrument, such as guitar, clarinet or drums, try moving your body with the rhythm.
5. Make a special dance-inspiring list of songs for long walks, hikes or other exercise where you can swing your arms, bop your head or move freely other ways in time to music.
6. When throwing yourself into a do-it-yourself project, such as painting a room, turn on music and get shaking.
7. If you're cooking or baking something that excites you, such as a favorite cake, add a heaping spoonful of boogie-down.

Happiness Upgrade Journal

*Give yourself a Happiness Upgrade, then note where you rank
on a happiness scale of 1 to 10 before and after.*

Date _____

Happiness Upgrades   before   after

_____   ○   ○

_____   ○   ○

_____   ○   ○

Date _____

Happiness Upgrades   before   after

_____   ○   ○

_____   ○   ○

_____   ○   ○

Date _____

Happiness Upgrades   before   after

_____   ○   ○

_____   ○   ○

_____   ○   ○

Date _____

Happiness Upgrades   before   after

_____   ○   ○

_____   ○   ○

_____   ○   ○

Date _____

Happiness Upgrades   before   after

_____   ○   ○

_____   ○   ○

_____   ○   ○

Date _____

Happiness Upgrades   before   after

_____   ○   ○

_____   ○   ○

_____   ○   ○

Date _____

Happiness Upgrades   before   after

_____   ○   ○

_____   ○   ○

_____   ○   ○

Default
Happiness Level

Happiness Upgrade:
Boost Caffeine With Sunshine

If you drink caffeinated beverages, such as coffee or black tea, great news: You can give your kickstart-in-a-cup a **Happiness Upgrade** by sipping it in a sunny spot. A study in the journal *Psychopharmacology* shows that combining caffeine and sunlight leads to a substantially bigger mood boost than drinking the same beverage in a dim setting or indoors under artificial light.[1]

Why it works

On their own, caffeine and sunlight are both mood-boosters: Caffeine increases good feelings by prompting a rise in dopamine and adrenaline; the sun's blue wavelength light increases mood-regulating serotonin. When combined, sunlight enhances caffeine-related changes in the brain, intensifying its happiness-lifting potency.

Happiness Upgrade suggestions:

1. Sip your brew on your front stoop, balcony or sunny porch.
2. Bring your lunch outside and pair it with a refreshing caffeinated beverage.
3. Head outdoors with your drink even if there are clouds in the sky since some of the sun's rays still reach you.
4. Stick to the sunny side of the street when sipping on a walk.
5. When drinking indoors, open a window shade to let the sun shine in or find a sunny spot, for instance, under a skylight.
6. If you're on public transportation with your travel mug, try finding a sun-drenched seat to settle into.
7. If you're in an area with little sunlight, consider getting a light bulb that casts blue wave light to mimic the sun's rays.

Happiness Upgrade Journal

Give yourself a Happiness Upgrade, then note where you rank on a happiness scale of 1 to 10 before and after.

Date _____

Happiness Upgrades　　before　after

_____　○　○

_____　○　○

_____　○　○

Date _____

Happiness Upgrades　　before　after

_____　○　○

_____　○　○

_____　○　○

Date _____

Happiness Upgrades　　before　after

_____　○　○

_____　○　○

_____　○　○

Date _____

Happiness Upgrades　　before　after

_____　○　○

_____　○　○

_____　○　○

Date _____

Happiness Upgrades　　before　after

_____　○　○

_____　○　○

_____　○　○

Date _____

Happiness Upgrades　　before　after

_____　○　○

_____　○　○

_____　○　○

Date _____

Happiness Upgrades　　before　after

_____　○　○

_____　○　○

_____　○　○

Default
Happiness Level

Happiness Upgrade:
Adopt a "Happy" Walking Style

You can give any walk you take a **Happiness Upgrade** by adopting a playful gait, such as swinging your arms like a kid with each step. A study in the *Journal of Behavior Therapy and Experimental Psychiatry* found that the way you walk impacts the way you feel—with a slumping, slow saunter bringing down your mood and an upright, jaunty stroll bringing it up.[1]

Why it works

Physical movements that you associate with being happy tell your brain that you're experiencing joy, so it unlocks uplifting memories to match this feeling. As a result, you recall more positive moments from the past, such as a visit to an amusement park or learning how to ride a bike. These happy recollections then fill you with cheer.

Happiness Upgrade suggestions:

1. Stand up straighter with your chin up, chest out and shoulders back.
2. Swing your arms up and down.
3. Speed up.
4. Meander in random directions rather than go straight ahead.
5. Bounce a little with each step.
6. Shimmy, shake or dance as you walk.
7. Skip!

Happiness Upgrade Journal

Give yourself a Happiness Upgrade, then note where you rank on a happiness scale of 1 to 10 before and after.

Date _____

Happiness Upgrades before after

_____ ○ ○
_____ ○ ○
_____ ○ ○

Date _____

Happiness Upgrades before after

_____ ○ ○
_____ ○ ○
_____ ○ ○

Date _____

Happiness Upgrades before after

_____ ○ ○
_____ ○ ○
_____ ○ ○

Date _____

Happiness Upgrades before after

_____ ○ ○
_____ ○ ○
_____ ○ ○

Date _____

Happiness Upgrades before after

_____ ○ ○
_____ ○ ○
_____ ○ ○

Date _____

Happiness Upgrades before after

_____ ○ ○
_____ ○ ○
_____ ○ ○

Date _____

Happiness Upgrades before after

_____ ○ ○
_____ ○ ○
_____ ○ ○

Default Happiness Level

Happiness Upgrade:
Pamper Yourself

When you have time where you won't be interrupted by people, pets, phones, emails, texts or anything else, give yourself a **Happiness Upgrade** by indulging in a session of self-pampering. This can be any beauty, grooming or wellness treatment you enjoy that you can do at home or have professionally done for you. Regularly setting aside "me-time" to improve your appearance or well-being ticks up joy in the present and also makes you less likely to develop depression in the future, shows a study in the journal *Health Psychology Research*.[1]

Why it works

Allowing time for self-pampering where you're focusing solely on yourself helps you escape daily stressors that weigh you down. It also increases self-esteem by reminding you that you're important and worth the extra-special care.

Happiness Upgrade suggestions:

1. Treat yourself to the kind of grooming that makes you feel better about yourself, such as a fresh shave or manicure.
2. Turn your shower into a spa indulgence by using salt scrubs, aromatic cleansers or an exfoliating brush.
3. Apply a homemade or store-bought hair conditioning treatment.
4. Take a luxurious soak with bath bombs or bubbles.
5. Get a relaxing massage from a professional massage therapist or use aromatic massage oil to rub your arms, calves, feet and hands.
6. Enjoy a do-it-yourself facial at home.
7. Book an appointment for a professional pampering session (for example, getting a haircut) that you've been putting off due to work, kids, caretaking or other responsibilities.

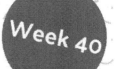

Happiness Upgrade Journal

Give yourself a Happiness Upgrade, then note where you rank on a happiness scale of 1 to 10 before and after.

Date _____
Happiness Upgrades before after
_____ ◯ ◯
_____ ◯ ◯
_____ ◯ ◯

Date _____
Happiness Upgrades before after
_____ ◯ ◯
_____ ◯ ◯
_____ ◯ ◯

Date _____
Happiness Upgrades before after
_____ ◯ ◯
_____ ◯ ◯
_____ ◯ ◯

Date _____
Happiness Upgrades before after
_____ ◯ ◯
_____ ◯ ◯
_____ ◯ ◯

Date _____
Happiness Upgrades before after
_____ ◯ ◯
_____ ◯ ◯
_____ ◯ ◯

Date _____
Happiness Upgrades before after
_____ ◯ ◯
_____ ◯ ◯
_____ ◯ ◯

Date _____
Happiness Upgrades before after
_____ ◯ ◯
_____ ◯ ◯
_____ ◯ ◯

Default
Happiness Level

Happiness Upgrade:
Add Fun to Your Workout

Love the mood lift you get from exercising? You can give yourself a **Happiness Upgrade** by pairing your workout with another activity you enjoy, such as listening to music or watching a movie. You'll experience greater pleasure than doing either alone, shows a study in *Journal of Sports Science & Medicine*.[1]

Why it works

Exercise is already proven to boost positivity, which scientists suspect is due in part to the release of happiness-enhancing endorphins and norepinephrine. When you add a fun activity to your workout, it distracts you from the boredom of repetitive movements and helps you forget about minor aches so you can focus more on the uplifting effects.

Happiness Upgrade suggestions:

1. Listen to your favorite music to match the pace of your exercise, for example, hard-driving tunes for fast or intense workouts.
2. Cue up a movie, TV show or video to watch during stationary workouts, such as on treadmills or indoor bikes.
3. Invite a pal to join you and enjoy chit-chat, swap workout tips, act as spotters or cheer each other on to go further.
4. Enjoy the latest episode of a favorite podcast or use the opportunity to discover to new podcasts.
5. Borrow audio versions of biographies, fiction, mysteries, self-help and other subjects from your library and listen as you work out.
6. Learn something new as you exercise, for example, attend a webinar or watch an instructional video.
7. Call a friend or family member during low-intensity workouts, such as walks, to catch up.

Happiness Upgrade Journal

*Give yourself a Happiness Upgrade, then note where you rank
on a happiness scale of 1 to 10 before and after.*

Date _____

Happiness Upgrades   before   after

_____   ○ ○
_____   ○ ○
_____   ○ ○

Date _____

Happiness Upgrades   before   after

_____   ○ ○
_____   ○ ○
_____   ○ ○

Date _____

Happiness Upgrades   before   after

_____   ○ ○
_____   ○ ○
_____   ○ ○

Date _____

Happiness Upgrades   before   after

_____   ○ ○
_____   ○ ○
_____   ○ ○

Date _____

Happiness Upgrades   before   after

_____   ○ ○
_____   ○ ○
_____   ○ ○

Date _____

Happiness Upgrades   before   after

_____   ○ ○
_____   ○ ○
_____   ○ ○

Date _____

Happiness Upgrades   before   after

_____   ○ ○
_____   ○ ○
_____   ○ ○

Default
Happiness Level

Happiness Upgrade:
Switch Off After Work

After a day when you've experienced high stress from work (such as tight deadlines) or due to home responsibilities (such as taking care of a child or parent), you can give yourself a **Happiness Upgrade** by taking at least 10 minutes to do an enjoyable activity that completely absorbs your attention. Research shows that this short amount of "switching off" replenishes positivity right away. An added plus: It makes you more upbeat when returning to your job or home commitments the following day.[1]

Why it works

Totally immersing yourself in a pleasant activity that you choose directs your attention away from work and daily responsibilities so you can fully disengage. This gives you a mental break that stops you from churning over worries, hassles or negative events you experienced during the day, which halts stress and resets your emotions.

Happiness Upgrade suggestions:

1. Enjoy a favorite hobby, such as creating art or gardening.
2. Treat yourself to entertainment, such as reading a book, playing a video game or watching a funny video.
3. Relax with yoga, meditation, tai chi or gentle stretching.
4. Get moving with a walk, jog, bike ride, swim or other exercise.
5. Catch up on the latest posts in an online discussion group you belong to.
6. Take your dog for a stroll, play with your cat or interact with another animal friend.
7. Do something nice for yourself, such as visit your favorite bakery or give your hair a deep conditioning treatment.

Happiness Upgrade Journal

Give yourself a Happiness Upgrade, then note where you rank on a happiness scale of 1 to 10 before and after.

Date _____
Happiness Upgrades   before   after
_____   ○   ○
_____   ○   ○
_____   ○   ○

Date _____
Happiness Upgrades   before   after
_____   ○   ○
_____   ○   ○
_____   ○   ○

Date _____
Happiness Upgrades   before   after
_____   ○   ○
_____   ○   ○
_____   ○   ○

Date _____
Happiness Upgrades   before   after
_____   ○   ○
_____   ○   ○
_____   ○   ○

Date _____
Happiness Upgrades   before   after
_____   ○   ○
_____   ○   ○
_____   ○   ○

Date _____
Happiness Upgrades   before   after
_____   ○   ○
_____   ○   ○
_____   ○   ○

Date _____
Happiness Upgrades   before   after
_____   ○   ○
_____   ○   ○
_____   ○   ○

Default Happiness Level

Happiness Upgrade:
Invest in Experiences

Want to buy something for yourself as a mood-boosting treat? You can give yourself an even bigger **Happiness Upgrade** by spending your cash on an experience rather than a material item. A study in *Journal of Experimental Social Psychology* found that folks who bought tickets to events, dined at restaurants or purchased other experiences were happier than those who spent money on products, such as jewelry and clothing.[1]

Why it works

The pleasure you get from material goods fades quickly. By comparison, experiences involve more senses, emotions and action so they leave lasting memories. Plus, they can add new skills or improve existing talents, which increases self-worth. You're also more likely to share what you experience with others, which can help foster relationships—another key way to kindle joy.

Happiness Upgrade suggestions:

1. Purchase tickets for an event that's unique or available only for a limited time, such as a band's one-night appearance.
2. Visit a restaurant that's special to you, for example, because it's where you celebrated after graduating school.
3. Take a trip to an interesting destination or visit a loved one.
4. Assemble an at-home date with yourself or with a pal, such as a do-it-yourself spa experience or movie night.
5. Buy an item that enables you to have an experience, such as a bicycle, kite, knitting kit or snorkel.
6. Sign up for lessons in cooking, painting or another subject to learn something new or advance skills you already have.
7. Invest in an experience that makes your life better, for example, consult with a registered dietitian to find out how to eat healthier.

Happiness Upgrade Journal

*Give yourself a Happiness Upgrade, then note where you rank
on a happiness scale of 1 to 10 before and after.*

Date _____

Happiness Upgrades   before after
_____
_____
_____

Date _____

Happiness Upgrades   before after
_____
_____
_____

Date _____

Happiness Upgrades   before after
_____
_____
_____

Date _____

Happiness Upgrades   before after
_____
_____
_____

Date _____

Happiness Upgrades   before after
_____
_____
_____

Date _____

Happiness Upgrades   before after
_____
_____
_____

Date _____

Happiness Upgrades   before after
_____
_____
_____

Default
Happiness Level

Happiness Upgrade:
Lend a Helping Hand

Offering to help a family member, friend, neighbor, classmate, stranger or other person is a surefire way to lift their spirits *and* it gives you an immediate **Happiness Upgrade**, too.[1] What's more, you'll get a bump in positivity even if you're currently dealing with your own stress or difficult challenges. The proof: In a study published in the journal *Culture and Brain*, researchers discovered that healthcare workers who volunteered to assist ailing patients during the height of the COVID-19 pandemic experienced extreme stress, however, they also reported greater happiness than folks who weren't volunteering.[2]

Why it works

Helping folks gives your life meaning, makes you feel more connected to others, increases your appreciation of times when people are kind to you and puts your own problems into perspective, making them seem more manageable.

Happiness Upgrade suggestions:

1. Bring food to a person, family or organization.
2. Give away items you don't need, such as books, clothing, electronics or furniture.
3. Offer to drive or arrange transportation for someone who needs to go to a doctor or other important destination.
4. Volunteer to write a review of a friend's book, music or business to help their endeavors grow.
5. Rake the yard of someone who is ill, injured or has a health challenge.
6. Visit someone who doesn't get to see people as often as they want, such as an elderly neighbor.
7. Ask someone what you could do to help.

Happiness Upgrade Journal

*Give yourself a Happiness Upgrade, then note where you rank
on a happiness scale of 1 to 10 before and after.*

Date _____

Happiness Upgrades before after
_____ ◯ ◯
_____ ◯ ◯
_____ ◯ ◯

Date _____

Happiness Upgrades before after
_____ ◯ ◯
_____ ◯ ◯
_____ ◯ ◯

Date _____

Happiness Upgrades before after
_____ ◯ ◯
_____ ◯ ◯
_____ ◯ ◯

Date _____

Happiness Upgrades before after
_____ ◯ ◯
_____ ◯ ◯
_____ ◯ ◯

Date _____

Happiness Upgrades before after
_____ ◯ ◯
_____ ◯ ◯
_____ ◯ ◯

Date _____

Happiness Upgrades before after
_____ ◯ ◯
_____ ◯ ◯
_____ ◯ ◯

Date _____

Happiness Upgrades before after
_____ ◯ ◯
_____ ◯ ◯
_____ ◯ ◯

Default
Happiness Level

Happiness Upgrade:
Look at Photos of Happy Times

Find old photos of favorite friends (such as schoolmates) and fun experiences you've had (for example, a kayaking adventure), and put them all in one place. Then, take a peek whenever you need a **Happiness Upgrade**. Research shows that recalling pleasant people and events from your past gives you a lift in the present.[1]

Why it works

Savoring happy memories mentally transports you back in time, reigniting the same joy you had when the pictures were taken. An added plus: Focusing on positives in your past makes you less likely to ruminate about negatives from long ago. As a result, your memories of former times get rosier, which ratchets up good feelings now.

Happiness Upgrade suggestions:

1. Turn your computer desktop into a slideshow of happy photos from your past or attach pics to your refrigerator.
2. Place an uplifting photo from your past somewhere you can access it easily, for example, in your smartphone's media folder or in a desk drawer.
3. Frame a special photo from a former fun adventure and place it somewhere you'll see it during the day.
4. Create a decorative scrapbook of your favorite nostalgic shots.
5. Post favorite pics on social media and share a story about each.
6. Host an "old picture night" with friends and swap stories about your favorite snapshots.
7. Ask friends and family if they have more pictures from shared adventures that they can give you.

Happiness Upgrade Journal

*Give yourself a Happiness Upgrade, then note where you rank
on a happiness scale of 1 to 10 before and after.*

Date _____
Happiness Upgrades before after

Date _____
Happiness Upgrades before after

Date _____
Happiness Upgrades before after

Date _____
Happiness Upgrades before after

Date _____
Happiness Upgrades before after

Date _____
Happiness Upgrades before after

Date _____
Happiness Upgrades before after

Default
Happiness Level

Happiness Upgrade:
Get Creative

Do you have a creative passion, such as baking, gardening, knitting, painting, photography, playing an instrument or writing? No matter what your artistic ability or medium, getting creative gives you a **Happiness Upgrade** immediately and continues to buoy your mood all the way through the following day, according to a study in *The Journal of Positive Psychology*.[1]

Why it works

Being creative gives you an opportunity to express yourself, gain mastery in a skill, achieve goals, share your craft with others and experience a "flow" state where you become fully engrossed in an activity you find pleasurable. All of this makes you feel more engaged and gives your life more meaning, increasing joy.

Happiness Upgrade suggestions:

1. Pinpoint the most convenient, inspired or energetic time for you to enjoy your art, then set aside that time in your schedule so you don't skip it.
2. Look for ways to advance your skills in your chosen art, such as getting guidance from a teacher or watching a video.
3. Join a group of folks who enjoy the same kind of creative pursuits so you can encourage each other.
4. Plan an art project that you can share with loved ones or an audience.
5. Try experimenting with your craft so that you're expanding your art in some new way.
6. Consider entering your art in a competition.
7. Join forces and collaborate with another artist.

Happiness Upgrade Journal

*Give yourself a Happiness Upgrade, then note where you rank
on a happiness scale of 1 to 10 before and after.*

Date _____
Happiness Upgrades   before   after
○ ○
○ ○
○ ○

Date _____
Happiness Upgrades   before   after
○ ○
○ ○
○ ○

Date _____
Happiness Upgrades   before   after
○ ○
○ ○
○ ○

Date _____
Happiness Upgrades   before   after
○ ○
○ ○
○ ○

Date _____
Happiness Upgrades   before   after
○ ○
○ ○
○ ○

Date _____
Happiness Upgrades   before   after
○ ○
○ ○
○ ○

Date _____
Happiness Upgrades   before   after
○ ○
○ ○
○ ○

Default
Happiness Level

Happiness Upgrade:
Say "Thanks"

To nudge up your mood and increase patience in stressful situations, write down or think about reasons to feel grateful. No matter what spurs your gratitude, pondering these perks gives you a **Happiness Upgrade** right away, research shows.[1] An added bonus: Scientists have found that when you count your blessings on a regular basis, you feel more joyful, optimistic, motivated, resilient and satisfied with your life.[2]

Why it works

Reflecting on what you can feel thankful for takes your mind off problems you may be experiencing and pivots your thoughts to what's good in your life. It also prompts a pleasurable feeling by activating areas of the brain involved in experiencing reward.

Happiness Upgrade suggestions:

1. After waking, think of three reasons to feel grateful.
2. While getting ready for your day ahead, look in the mirror and tell yourself one thing you're thankful for.
3. Keep a written journal, dot graph "bullet" journal, scrapbook or video blog to celebrate all you appreciate.
4. Create or find artwork that reminds you to appreciate what's good, then put it where you'll see it regularly.
5. When you're in a stressful situation, pause to think about one silver lining. For example, if you're stuck in traffic, maybe you can appreciate that the radio is playing a favorite song.
6. Try to reflect on good fortune as it happens.
7. Before you fall asleep, pinpoint one or more moments in your day that made you glad.

Happiness Upgrade Journal

*Give yourself a Happiness Upgrade, then note where you rank
on a happiness scale of 1 to 10 before and after.*

Date _____

Happiness Upgrades   before   after

Date _____

Happiness Upgrades   before   after

Date _____

Happiness Upgrades   before   after

Date _____

Happiness Upgrades   before   after

Date _____

Happiness Upgrades   before   after

Date _____

Happiness Upgrades   before   after

Date _____

Happiness Upgrades   before   after

Default Happiness Level

Happiness Upgrade:
Talk More Deeply With a Buddy

Chatting with friends, family members, neighbors and strangers tends to make most folks happier, even if you consider yourself an introvert. But, you'll get an even bigger **Happiness Upgrade** from these talks when you bring up topics that are meaningful to you (such as a recent book you enjoyed) rather than sticking to superficial topics (like the weather), concludes a study in the journal *Psychological Science*.[1]

Why it works

Talking with others about anything has its own benefits: When you chat with favorite people, it strengthens your bonds with them. And, chatting with strangers gives you the sense of being tied to the community as a whole. In turn, these tighter connections make you feel supported and cared for, which increases self-esteem and confidence. So, it may be that when you bring up topics that are important to you to any of these folks, it gives the experience of connecting even more meaning, enhancing these positive emotions.

Happiness Upgrade suggestions:

1. Talk about a recent uplifting experience you've had, such as taking a class or attending a sporting event.
2. Swap details about recent books you've read, movies you've watched or podcasts you've listened to.
3. Share any recent triumphs you've achieved.
4. Pass along an interesting tidbit you recently learned.
5. Ask for advice on an issue you're dealing with.
6. Share details of an upcoming trip you're taking.
7. Recommend something you enjoy that you think someone else might, too, such as a favorite hobby.

Happiness Upgrade Journal

Give yourself a Happiness Upgrade, then note where you rank on a happiness scale of 1 to 10 before and after.

Date _____
Happiness Upgrades   before   after
_____   ○   ○
_____   ○   ○
_____   ○   ○

Date _____
Happiness Upgrades   before   after
_____   ○   ○
_____   ○   ○
_____   ○   ○

Date _____
Happiness Upgrades   before   after
_____   ○   ○
_____   ○   ○
_____   ○   ○

Date _____
Happiness Upgrades   before   after
_____   ○   ○
_____   ○   ○
_____   ○   ○

Date _____
Happiness Upgrades   before   after
_____   ○   ○
_____   ○   ○
_____   ○   ○

Date _____
Happiness Upgrades   before   after
_____   ○   ○
_____   ○   ○
_____   ○   ○

Date _____
Happiness Upgrades   before   after
_____   ○   ○
_____   ○   ○
_____   ○   ○

Default Happiness Level

Happiness Upgrade:
Stir Up Nostalgia

Most of us cherish at least some experiences from our past, whether it was from when we were kids, teens, young adults, young parents, early career-creators, ingénue artists or novice travelers of the world. If you take time to recreate one of these former experiences, you'll give yourself a **Happiness Upgrade** that leaves you beaming.

Why it works

Stirring up nostalgic memories reminds you of the loving connections you have with family and friends who are linked to those recollections. This increases self-esteem and makes you optimistic about your future, which are important ingredients for inner joy, say researchers from the United Kingdom's University of Southampton.[1].

Happiness Upgrade suggestions:

1. Enjoy entertainment that was a favorite from years ago, such as a kid's TV show you watched with your siblings.
2. Bake or cook a food that reminds you of homey comfort, such as the first meal you learned to make yourself.
3. Recreate a cherished tradition that you do for a holiday or other event.
4. Breathe in an aroma that reminds you of your grandparents' house, a trip you took or another happy experience.
5. Visit a store, restaurant, farmstand or other destination that's meaningful to you.
6. Head to an area of your town where you've had joy-filled experiences that you want to remember.
7. Call a family member or friend to swap stories about people, places or experiences you loved from the past.

Happiness Upgrade Journal

*Give yourself a Happiness Upgrade, then note where you rank
on a happiness scale of 1 to 10 before and after.*

Date _____

Happiness Upgrades before after

_____

Date _____

Happiness Upgrades before after

_____

Date _____

Happiness Upgrades before after

_____

Date _____

Happiness Upgrades before after

_____

Date _____

Happiness Upgrades before after

_____

Date _____

Happiness Upgrades before after

_____

Date _____

Happiness Upgrades before after

_____

Default
Happiness Level

Happiness Upgrade:
Touch Something Soft

Sounds too silly to work, but getting a **Happiness Upgrade** can be as easy as touching something soft.

Why it works

Feeling soft, fuzzy or squishy textures against your skin triggers pleasant emotions, shows a study in the journal *Consciousness and Cognition*.[1] Why? Over time, your brain becomes trained to associate soft surfaces with enjoyable experiences, for example, furry cats and mushy pillows. So, every time you feel a similar texture, it produces a happy feeling.

Happiness Upgrade suggestions:

1. Walk barefoot on grass, sand, a thick rug or other soft surfaces.
2. Pet a cat, dog, hamster or other furry creature.
3. Hug a plush toy or curl up on the couch with a fuzzy blanket.
4. Keep a squishy ball nearby to squeeze.
5. Wear clothing made of material known for its softness, such as fleece and jersey.
6. Don extra cushy socks or slippers.
7. Add smushy pillows to a chair or couch.

Happiness Upgrade Journal

Give yourself a Happiness Upgrade, then note where you rank on a happiness scale of 1 to 10 before and after.

Date _____
Happiness Upgrades　　before　after
_____ ○ ○
_____ ○ ○
_____ ○ ○

Date _____
Happiness Upgrades　　before　after
_____ ○ ○
_____ ○ ○
_____ ○ ○

Date _____
Happiness Upgrades　　before　after
_____ ○ ○
_____ ○ ○
_____ ○ ○

Date _____
Happiness Upgrades　　before　after
_____ ○ ○
_____ ○ ○
_____ ○ ○

Date _____
Happiness Upgrades　　before　after
_____ ○ ○
_____ ○ ○
_____ ○ ○

Date _____
Happiness Upgrades　　before　after
_____ ○ ○
_____ ○ ○
_____ ○ ○

Date _____
Happiness Upgrades　　before　after
_____ ○ ○
_____ ○ ○
_____ ○ ○

Default Happiness Level

Happiness Upgrade:
Learn to Do One Thing Better

Have a hobby, skill or talent that you enjoy, for example, playing a musical instrument or cooking? You can use it to get a **Happiness Upgrade** by learning one new way to be better at it, for example, you might learn a new fill on the drums or how to caramelize onions. Even if it's just a small improvement, you'll get a spike in good feelings.

Why it works

Advancing your skill has a variety of mood-lifting effects on you: Mastering a new aspect of a pleasurable activity increases how much you enjoy it, plus it boosts self-esteem by making you feel more capable. Continuing to learn adds meaning to your life and gives you a sense of purpose. And, learning anything new spurs the release of feel-good dopamine in the brain.[1]

Happiness Upgrade suggestions:

1. Bookmark instructional websites, follow podcasts, subscribe to YouTube channels or get books about the activity you enjoy.
2. Sign up for a one-time webinar or an ongoing class.
3. Start an online discussion on social media about your interest to get input from other folks.
4. Join an in-person or online group dedicated to the activity.
5. Reach out to a friend, mentor or family member who shares the same passion and ask for their tips.
6. Ask a business owner, librarian or teacher to help you find out where professionals in the field you enjoy go to learn more about the subject.
7. Experiment with trying new techniques that you make up yourself. Keep notes as you do them to ensure you remember the ones that work.

Happiness Upgrade Journal

Give yourself a Happiness Upgrade, then note where you rank
on a happiness scale of 1 to 10 before and after.

Date _____
Happiness Upgrades before after
_____ ○ ○
_____ ○ ○
_____ ○ ○

Date _____
Happiness Upgrades before after
_____ ○ ○
_____ ○ ○
_____ ○ ○

Date _____
Happiness Upgrades before after
_____ ○ ○
_____ ○ ○
_____ ○ ○

Date _____
Happiness Upgrades before after
_____ ○ ○
_____ ○ ○
_____ ○ ○

Date _____
Happiness Upgrades before after
_____ ○ ○
_____ ○ ○
_____ ○ ○

Date _____
Happiness Upgrades before after
_____ ○ ○
_____ ○ ○
_____ ○ ○

Date _____
Happiness Upgrades before after
_____ ○ ○
_____ ○ ○
_____ ○ ○

Default Happiness Level

Happiness Upgrade:
Take a 5-Minute Waking Rest Break

In today's go-go-go world, doing absolutely nothing may seem like wasted time. However, sitting or lying quietly without doing anything else for 5 to 20 minutes while awake can give you a **Happiness Upgrade** that nudges up good feelings, making it easier to move on with the rest of your day.[1] Called "waking rest", your eyes can be open or closed and you simply let your thoughts wander wherever they want without judging them.

Why it works

Researchers suspect this time-out technique improves mood by giving you an opportunity to relax as well as to pause the constant influx of stimulation, which replenishes mental energy.

Happiness Upgrade suggestions:

1. Create a comfortable spot to use as your regular "waking rest" place, such as a relaxing chair.
2. Take a waking rest break during or after a task that requires lots of brainwork, such as coding, reading or writing.
3. After you've completed a long or strenuous task, take a waking rest break before putting on TV, music, video games or another form of media.
4. Every once in a while, treat yourself to a new spot for a waking rest period, such as your bathtub or a park bench.
5. Use waking rest when traveling, for example, to unwind from a flight or decompress during or after a day full of activities.
6. If doing waking rest with your eyes open, experiment with different locations to direct your gaze, such as the night sky.
7. Add a specific time in your daily calendar for waking rest or set a timer so you can remember to do it.

Happiness Upgrade Journal

*Give yourself a Happiness Upgrade, then note where you rank
on a happiness scale of 1 to 10 before and after.*

Date _____
Happiness Upgrades   before   after
_____
_____
_____

Date _____
Happiness Upgrades   before   after
_____
_____
_____

Date _____
Happiness Upgrades   before   after
_____
_____
_____

Date _____
Happiness Upgrades   before   after
_____
_____
_____

Date _____
Happiness Upgrades   before   after
_____
_____
_____

Date _____
Happiness Upgrades   before   after
_____
_____
_____

Date _____
Happiness Upgrades   before   after
_____
_____
_____

Default
Happiness Level

Endnotes

Chapter 1

[1] Jessie Hackford, Anna Mackey, Elizabeth Broadbent, "The Effects of Walking Posture on Affective and Physiological States During Stress", *Journal of Behavior Therapy and Experimental Psychiatry*, 62 (2019): 80-87
Carissa Wilkes, et al., "Upright Posture Improves Affect and Fatigue in People With Depressive Symptoms", *Journal of Behavior Therapy and Experimental Psychiatry*, 54 (2017): 143-149

[2] Lowry. A. Kirkby, et al., "An Amygdala-Hippocampus Subnetwork that Encodes Variation in Human Mood", *Cell*, 175 (2018): P1688-1700
Elizabeth A. Kensinger, "Negative Emotion Enhances Memory Accuracy: Behavioral and Neuroimaging Evidence", *Current Directions in Psychological Science*, published online August 1, 2007

[3] Barbara L. Fredrickson, "What Good Are Positive Emotions?", *Review of General Psychology*, 2 (1998): 300-319
Barbara L. Fredrickson, "The Role of Positive Emotions in Positive Psychology. The Broaden-and-Build Theory of Positive Emotions", *The American Psychologist*, 56 (2001): 218-226

[4] Andrea B. Burns, et al., "Upward Spirals of Positive Emotion and Coping: Replication, Extension, and Initial Exploration of Neurochemical Substrates", *Personality and Individual Differences*, 44 (2008): 360-370
Barbara L. Fredrickson, Thomas Joiner, "Positive Emotions Trigger Upward Spirals Toward Emotional Well-Being", *Psychological Science*, 13 (2002): 172-175

[5] Michael A. Cohn, et al., "Happiness Unpacked: Positive Emotions Increase Life Satisfaction by Building Resilience", *Emotion*, 9 (2009): 361-368

[6] Kristin Layous, et al., "Delivering Happiness: Translating Positive Psychology Intervention Research for Treating Major and Minor Depressive Disorders", *Journal of Alternative and Complementary Medicine*, 17 (2011): 675-683
Nancy L. Sin, Sonja Lyubomirsky, "Enhancing Well-Being and Alleviating Depressive Symptoms with Positive Psychology Interventions: A Practice-Friendly Meta-Analysis", *Journal of Clinical Psychology*, 65 (2009): 467-487

[7] Beatriz Pereira, Scott Rick, "Why Retail Therapy Works: It Is Choice, Not Acquisition, That Primarily Alleviates Sadness", *The Association for Consumer Research*, 39 (2011): 732-733

[8] Hannah Raila, Brian J. Scholl, June Gruber, "Seeing the World Through Rose-Colored Glasses: People Who Are Happy and Satisfied with Life Preferentially Attend to Positive Stimuli", *Emotion*, 15 (2015): 449-462

[9] Eni S. Becker, et al., "Always Approach the Bright Side of Life: A General Positivity Training Reduces Stress Reactions in Vulnerable Individuals", *Cognitive Therapy and Research*, published online September 25, 2015

[10] Mark A. Thompson, et al., "Pleasant Emotions Widen Thought-Action Repertoires, Develop Long-Term Resources, and Improve Reaction Time Performance: A Multi-Study Examination of the Broaden-and-Build Theory Among Athletes", *Journal of Sport & Exercise Psychology*, 43 (2021): 155-170

Chapter 3

[1] Takaaki Ozawa, et al., "A Feedback Neural Circuit for Calibrating Aversive Memory Strength", *Nature Neuroscience*, 20 (2017): 90-97
Elizabeth A. Kensinger, "Negative Emotion Enhances Memory Accuracy: Behavioral and Neuroimaging Evidence", *Current Directions in Psychological Science*, published online August 1, 2007

[2] Barbara L. Fredrickson, Cara Arizmendi, Patty Van Cappellen, "Same-Day, Cross-Day, and Upward Spiral Relations Between Positive Affect and Positive Health Behaviours", *Psychology & Health*, 36 (2021): 444-460
Patty Van Cappellen, et al., "Positive Affective Processes Underlie Positive Health Behaviour Change", *Psychology & Health*, 33 (2018): 77-97
Mohammad Siahpush, Matt Spittal, Gopal K. Singh, "Happiness and Life Satisfaction Prospectively Predict Self-Rated Health, Physical Health, and the Presence of Limiting, Long-Term Health Conditions", *American Journal of Health Promotion*, 23 (2008): 18-26

Chapter 4

[1] David Lykken, Auke Tellegen, "Happiness is a Stochastic Phenomenon", *Psychological Science*, 7 (1996): 186-189
Bruce Headey, Alexander Wearing, "Personality, Life Events, and Subjective Well-Being: Toward a Dynamic Equilibrium Model", *Journal of Personality and Social Psychology*, 57 (1989): 731–739
Philip Brickman, Donald T. Campbell. 1971. "Hedonic Relativism and Planning the Good Science", *Adaptation-Level Theory: A Symposium*, edited by Mortimer Herbert Appley, 287–302, Academic Press

[2] Bruce Headey, Ruud Muffels, Gert G. Wagner, "Long-Running German Panel Survey Shows That Personal and Economic Choices, Not Just Genes, Matter

for Happiness", *Proceedings of the National Academy of Sciences*, 107 (2010): 17922-17926

52-Week Journal

Week 1

[1] Dacher Keltner, Richard Bowman, Harriet Richards, "Exploring the Emotional State of 'Real Happiness': A Study Into the Effects of Watching Natural History Television Content", The Real Happiness Project, British Broadcast Company's (BBC), 2017, RealHappinessProject.org
Richard M. Ryan, et al., "Vitalizing Effects of Being Outdoors and in Nature", *Journal of Environmental Psychology*, 30 (2010): 159-168

Week 2

[1] Christopher K. Hsee, Adelle X. Yang, Liangyan Wang, "Idleness Aversion and the Need for Justifiable Busyness", *Psychological Science*, 21 (2010): 926-930

Week 3

[1] Aaron S. Heller, et al., "Association Between Real-World Experiential Diversity and Positive Affect Relates to Hippocampal-Striatal Functional Connectivity", *Nature Neuroscience*, 23 (2020): 800–804
Thomas E. Hazy, Michael J. Frank, Randall C. O'Reilly, "Neural Mechanisms of Acquired Phasic Dopamine Responses in Learning", *Neuroscience & Biobehavioral Reviews*, 34 (2010): 701-720
Nico Bunzeck, Emrah Düzel, "Absolute Coding of Stimulus Novelty in the Human Substantia Nigra/VTA", *Neuron*, 51 (2006): 369-379
Sham Kakade, Peter Dayan, "Dopamine: Generalization and Bonuses", *Neural Networks*, 15 (2002): 549-559

Week 4

[1] Tomohiro Ishizu, Semir Zeki, "Toward a Brain-Based Theory of Beauty", *PLOS ONE*, 6 (2011): e21852

Week 5

[1] Jaap J. A. Denissen, et al., "The Effects of Weather on Daily Mood: A Multilevel Approach", *Emotion*, 8 (2008): 662– 667
Craig A. Anderson, et al., "Temperature and Aggression", *Advances in Experimental Social Psychology*, 32 (2000): 63-133

Douglas T. Kenrick, Steven W. MacFarlane, "Ambient Temperature and Horn Honking: A Field Study of the Heat/Aggression Relationship", *Environment and Behavior*, 18 (1986): 179-191

Week 6

[1] David G. Smith, et al., "Identification and Characterization of a Novel Anti-Inflammatory Lipid Isolated from *Mycobacterium Vaccae*, a Soil-Derived Bacterium with Immunoregulatory and Stress Resilience Properties", *Pscyhopharmacology*, 236 (2019): 1653–1670
Dorothy M. Matthews, Susan M. Jenks, "Ingestion of *Mycobacterium Vaccae* Decreases Anxiety-Related Behavior and Improves Learning in Mice", *Behavioural Processes*, 96 (2013): 27-35
Christopher A. Lowry, et al., "Identification of an Immune-Responsive Mesolimbocortical Serotonergic System: Potential Role in Regulation of Emotional Behavior", *Neuroscience*, 146 (2007): 756-772

[2] Jeannette Haviland-Jones, et al., "An Environmental Approach to Positive Emotion: Flowers", *Evolutionary Psychology*, 3 (2005): 104-132

[3] M. A. Leavell, et al., "Nature-Based Social Prescribing in Urban Settings to Improve Social Connectedness and Mental Well-Being: A Review", *Current Environmental Health Reports*, 6 (2019): 297-308
Agnes E. Van Den Berg, Mariëtte H.G. Custers, "Gardening Promotes Neuroendocrine and Affective Restoration from Stress", *Journal of Health Psychology*, 16 (2011): 3-11

Week 7

[1] Dan-Mikael Ellingsen, et al., "In Touch with Your Emotions: Oxytocin and Touch Change Social Impressions While Others' Facial Expressions Can Alter Touch", *Psychoneuroendocrinology*, 39 (2014): 11-20
Angeliki Theodoridou, et al., "Oxytocin and Social Perception: Oxytocin Increases Perceived Facial Trustworthiness and Attractiveness", *Hormones and Behavior*, 56 (2009): 128-132
Paul J. Zak, Angela A. Stanton, Sheila Ahmadi, "Oxytocin Increases Generosity in Humans", *PLOS ONE*, 2 (2007): e1128
Kathleen C. Light, Karen M. Grewen, Janet A. Amico, "More Frequent Partner Hugs and Higher Oxytocin Levels Are Linked to Lower Blood Pressure and Heart Rate in Premenopausal Women", *Biological Psychology*, 69 (2005): 5-21

Week 8

[1] Charlotte Fritz, et al., "Happy, Healthy, and Productive: The Role of Detachment from Work During Nonwork Time", *The Journal of Applied Psychology*, 95 (2010): 977-983

Week 9

[1] Valorie N. Salimpoor, et al., "Anatomically Distinct Dopamine Release During Anticipation and Experience of Peak Emotion to Music", *Nature Neuroscience*, 14 (2011): 257-262
Valorie N. Salimpoor, et al., "The Rewarding Aspects of Music Listening Are Related to Degree of Emotional Arousal", *PLOS ONE*, 4 (2009): e7487

Week 10

[1] Janine M. Dutcher, et al., "Self-Affirmation Activates the Ventral Striatum: A Possible Reward-Related Mechanism for Self-Affirmation", *Psychological Science*, 27 (2016): 455-66

Week 11

[1] Jolanda Jetten, et al., "Having a Lot of a Good Thing: Multiple Important Group Memberships as a Source of Self-Esteem", *PLOS ONE*, 10 (2015): e0124609

Week 12

[1] Andrew P. Allen, Andrew P. Smith, "Chewing Gum: Cognitive Performance, Mood, Well-Being, and Associated Physiology", *BioMed Research International*, published online May 17, 2015
Akiyo Sasaki-Otomaru, et al., "Effect of Regular Gum Chewing on Levels of Anxiety, Mood, and Fatigue in Healthy Young Adults", *Clinical Practice & Epidemiology in Mental Health*, 7 (2011): 133-139
Andrew Smith, "Effects of Chewing Gum on Cognitive Function, Mood and Physiology in Stressed and Non-Stressed Volunteers", *Nutritional Neuroscience*, 13 (2010): 7-16

[2] C. Philip Beaman, Kitty Powell, Ellie Rapley, "Want to Block Earworms from Conscious Awareness? B(u)y Gum!", *Quarterly Journal of Experimental Psychology*, 68 (2015): 1049-1057

Week 13

[1] Rebecca A. Blackie, Nancy L. Kocovski, "Letting Go of Yesterday: Effect of Distraction on Post-Event Processing and Anticipatory Anxiety in a Socially Anxious Sample", *Cognitive Behaviour Therapy*, 45 (2016): 60-72

Week 14

[1] Mirosław Karpiński, et al., "Effect of Stroking on Serotonin, Noradrenaline and Cortisol Levels in the Blood of Right- and Left-Pawed Dogs", *Animals*, 11 (2021): 331
Miho Nagasawa, et al., "Social evolution. Oxytocin-Gaze Positive Loop and the Co-Evolution of Human-Dog Bonds", *Science*, 348 (2015): 333-336
Linda Handlin, et al., "Short-Term Interaction between Dogs and Their Owners: Effects on Oxytocin, Cortisol, Insulin and Heart Rate—An Exploratory Study", Anthrozoös, 24 (2011): 301-315

[2] Karen Allen, Jim Blascovich, Wendy B. Mendes, "Cardiovascular Reactivity and the Presence of Pets, Friends, and Spouses: The Truth About Cats and Dogs", *Psychosomatic Medicine*, 64 (2002): 727-739

[3] Rebecca A. Johnson, Johannes S. J. Odendaal, Richard L. Meadows, "Animal-Assisted Interventions Research: Issues and Answers", *Western Journal of Nursing Research*, 24 (2002): 422-440

Week 15

[1] Edmund Keogh, et al. "The Effects of Menstrual-Related Pain on Attentional Interference," *Pain*, 155 (2014): 821-827
Ulrike Bingel, et al., "fMRI Reveals How Pain Modulates Visual Object Processing in the Ventral Visual Stream," *Neuron*, 55 (2007): 157-167
Chris Eccleston, Geert Crombez, "Pain Demands Attention: A Cognitive-Affective Model of the Interruptive Function of Pain," *Psychological Bulletin*, 125 (1999): 356-366

[2] Lisa Doan, Toby Manders, Jing Wang, "Neuroplasticity Underlying the Comorbidity of Pain and Depression", *Neural Plasticity*, published online February 25, 2015
Kimberly T. Sibille, et al., "Affect Balance Style, Experimental Pain Sensitivity, and Pain-Related Responses", *The Clinical Journal of Pain*, 28 (2012): 410-417
Michael Karl Boettger, Christiane Schwier, Karl-Jürgen Bär, "Sad Mood Increases Pain Sensitivity Upon Thermal Grill Illusion Stimulation: Implications for Central Pain Processing", *Pain*, 152 (2011): 123-130

Week 16

[1] Carolina Ramos Mendonça, et al., "Effects of Flavonols on Emotional Behavior and Compounds of the Serotonergic System: A Preclinical Systematic Review", *European Journal of Pharmacology*, 916 (2022): 174697

[2] Astrid Nehlig, Jean-Luc Daval, Gérard Debry, "Caffeine and the Central Nervous System: Mechanisms of Action, Biochemical, Metabolic and Psychostimulant Effects", *Brain Research Reviews*, 17 (1992): 139-170

[3] Natalie A. Masento, et al., "Effects of Hydration Status on Cognitive Performance and Mood", *The British Journal of Nutrition*, 111 (2014): 1841-1852
Lawrence E. Armstrong, et al., "Mild Dehydration Affects Mood in Healthy Young Women", *The Journal of Nutrition*, 142 (2012): 382-388
Matthew S. Ganio, et al., "Mild Dehydration Impairs Cognitive Performance and Mood of Men", *The British Journal of Nutrition*, (2011): 1535-1543

Week 17

[1] Jeroen Nawijn, et al., "Vacationers Happier, but Most Not Happier After a Holiday", *Applied Research in Quality of Life*, 5 (2010): 35-47

[2] Jan Packer, "Taking a Break: Exploring the Restorative Benefits of Short Breaks and Vacations", *Annals of Tourism Research Empirical Insights*, 2 (2021): 100006

Week 18

[1] Jennifer L. Trew, Lynn E. Alden, "Kindness Reduces Avoidance Goals in Socially Anxious Individuals", *Motivation and Emotion*, 39 (2015): 892-907

Week 19

[1] Ed O'Brien, Robert W. Smith, "Unconventional Consumption Methods and Enjoying Things Consumed: Recapturing the 'First-Time' Experience", *Personality and Social Psychology Bulletin*, 45 (2019): 67-80

Week 20

[1] Nicole L Stone, et al., "An Analysis of Endocannabinoid Concentrations and Mood Following Singing and Exercise in Healthy Volunteers", *Frontiers in Behavioral Neuroscience*, published online November 26, 2018
Norma Daykin, et al., "What Works for Well-Being? A Systematic Review of Well-Being Outcomes for Music and Singing in Adults", *Perspectives in Public Health*, 138 (2018): 39-46

[2] T. Moritz Schladt, "Choir Versus Solo Singing: Effects on Mood, and Salivary Oxytocin and Cortisol Concentrations", *Frontiers in Human Neuroscience*, published online September 14, 2017

Week 21

[1] Songlin Jiang, et al., "Effect of Fragrant Primula Flowers on Physiology and Psychology in Female College Students: An Empirical Study", *Frontiers in Psychology*, published online February 23, 2021

Kandhasamy Sowndhararajan, Songmun Kim, "Influence of Fragrances on Human Psychophysiological Activity: With Special Reference to Human Electroencephalographic Response", *Scientia Pharmaceutica*, 84 (2016): 724-752

Eijiro Fujii, et al., "Physiological and Psychological Response to Floral Scent", *HortScience*, 48 (2013): 82-88

Jeannette Haviland-Jones, et al., "The Emotional Air in Your Space: Scrubbed, Wild or Cultivated?", *Emotion, Space and Society*, 6 (2013): 91-99

Sandra T. Weber, Eva Heuberger, "The Impact of Natural Odors on Affective States in Humans", *Chemical Senses*, 33 (2008): 441-447

Week 22

[1] Ed O'Brien, Ellen Roney, "Worth the Wait? Leisure Can Be Just as Enjoyable With Work Left Undone", *Psychological Science*, 28 (2017): 1000-1015

Week 23

[1] Wändi Bruine de Bruin, Andrew M. Parker, JoNell Strough, "Choosing to be Happy? Age Differences in 'Maximizing' Decision Strategies and Experienced Emotional Well-Being", *Psychology and Aging*, 31 (2016): 295-300

Erin A. Sparks, Joyce Ehrlinger, Richard P. Eibach, "Failing to Commit: Maximizers Avoid Commitment in a Way That Contributes to Reduced Satisfaction", *Personality and Individual Differences*, 52 (2012): 72-77

Week 24

[1] Barbara Wild, et al., "Why Are Smiles Contagious? An fMRI study of the Interaction Between Perception of Facial Affect and Facial Movements", *Psychiatry Research*, 123 (2003): 17-36

Week 25

[1] Norris F. Krueger, Peter R. Dickson, "How Believing in Ourselves Increases Risk Taking: Perceived Self-Efficacy and Opportunity Recognition", *Decision Sciences*, 25 (2007): 385-400

Todd B. Kashdan, Michael F. Steger, "Curiosity and Pathways to Well-Being and Meaning in Life: Traits, States, and Everyday Behaviors", *Motivation and Emotion*, 31 (2007): 159-173

Thomas Dohmen, et al., "Individual Risk Attitudes: New Evidence From a Large, Representative, Experimentally Validated Survey", *Journal of the European Economic Association*, Discussion Papers 511, September 2005

[2] Milky Kohno, et al., "Risk-Taking Behavior: Dopamine D2/D3 Receptors, Feedback, and Frontolimbic Activity", *Cerebral Cortex*, 25 (2015): 236–245

[3] Beatriz Pereira, Scott Rick, "Why Retail Therapy Works: It Is Choice, Not Acquisition, That Primarily Alleviates Sadness", *The Association for Consumer Research*, 39 (2011): 732-733

Week 26

[1] Lysann Damisch, Barbara Stoberock, Thomas Mussweiler, "Keep Your Fingers Crossed!: How Superstition Improves Performance", *Psychological Science*, 21 (2010): 1014-1020
Liza Day, John Maltby, "Belief in Good Luck and Psychological Well-Being: The Mediating Role of Optimism and Irrational Beliefs", *The Journal of Psychology*, 137 (2003): 99-110

Week 27

[1] Julia C. Basso, Wendy A. Suzuki, "The Effects of Acute Exercise on Mood, Cognition, Neurophysiology, and Neurochemical Pathways: A Review", *Brain Plasticity*, 2 (2017): 127-152
Justy Reed, Deniz S. Ones, "The Effect of Acute Aerobic Exercise on Positive Activated Affect: A Meta-Analysis", *Psychology of Sport and Exercise*, 7 (2006): 477-514
Bonnie G. Berger, David R. Owen, "Relation of Low and Moderate Intensity Exercise with Acute Mood Change in College Joggers", *Perceptual and Motor Skills*, 87 (1998): 611-621
Emmanuel Maroulakis, Yannis Zervas, "Effects of Aerobic Exercise on Mood of Adult Women", *Perceptual and Motor Skills*, 76 (1993): 795-801

[2] Lauren E. Salcia, Kathleen A. Martin Ginis, "Acute Effects of Exercise on Women With Pre-existing Body Image Concerns: A Test of Potential Mediators", *Psychology of Sport and Exercise*, 31 (2017): 113-122
Naomi J. Ellis, Jason A. Randall, Grant Punnett, "The Effects of a Single Bout of Exercise on Mood and Self-Esteem in Clinically Diagnosed Mental Health Patients", *Open Journal of Medical Psychology*, 2 (2013): 81-85

Week 28

[1] Elaine Hatfield, et al., "New Perspectives on Emotional Contagion: A Review of Classic and Recent Research on Facial Mimicry and Contagion",

Interpersona: An International Journal on Personal Relationships, 8 (2014): 159-179

Mary J. Howes, Jack E. Hokanson, David A. Loewenstein, "Induction of Depressive Affect After Prolonged Exposure to a Mildly Depressed Individual", *Journal of Personality and Social Psychology*, 49 (1985): 1110-1113

Week 29

[1] Jia Wei Zhang, Serena Chen, Teodora K. Tomova Shakur, "From Me to You: Self-Compassion Predicts Acceptance of Own and Others' Imperfections", *Personality & Social Psychology Bulletin*, 46 (2020): 228-242

Madeleine Ferrari, et al., "Self-Compassion Moderates the Perfectionism and Depression Link in Both Adolescence and Adulthood", *PLOS ONE*, 13 (2018): e0192022

Katie E. Gunnell, et al. "Don't Be So Hard on Yourself! Changes in Self-Compassion During the First Year of University Are Associated With Changes in Well-Being", *Personality and Individual Differences*, 107 (2017): 43-48

Week 30

[1] Liudmila Titova, Kennon M. Sheldon, "Happiness Comes From Trying to Make Others Feel Good, Rather Than Oneself", *The Journal of Positive Psychology*, published March 8, 2021

Soyoung Q. Park, et al., "A Neural Link Between Generosity and Happiness", *Nature Communications*, 8 (2017): 15964

Elizabeth B. Raposa, Holly B. Laws, Emily B. Ansell, "Prosocial Behavior Mitigates the Negative Effects of Stress in Everyday Life", *Clinical Psychological Science*, 4 (2016): 691-698

S. Katherine Nelson, et al., "Do Unto Others or Treat Yourself? The Effects of Prosocial and Self-Focused Behavior on Psychological Flourishing", *Emotion*, 16 (2016): 850–861

Elizabeth W. Dunn, Lara B. Aknin, Michael I. Norton, "Prosocial Spending and Happiness: Using Money to Benefit Others Pays Off", *Current Directions in Psychological Science*, published online February 3, 2014

Kathryn E. Buchanan, Anat Bardi, "Acts of Kindness and Acts of Novelty Affect Life Satisfaction", *The Journal of Social Psychology*, 150 (2010): 235-237

Week 31

[1] Ed O'Brien, Phoebe C. Ellsworth, "Saving the Last for Best: A Positivity Bias for End Experiences", *Psychological Science*, 23 (2012): 163-165

Week 32

[1] Pablo Briñol, et al., "Treating Thoughts as Material Objects Can Increase or Decrease Their Impact on Evaluation", *Psychological Science*, 24 (2013): 41-47

Week 33

[1] Jeffrey Conrath Miller, Zlatan Krizan, "Walking Facilitates Positive Affect (Even When Expecting the Opposite)", *Emotion*, 16 (2016): 775-785

Week 34

[1] Desirée Colombo, et al., "Savoring the Present: The Reciprocal Influence Between Positive Emotions and Positive Emotion Regulation in Everyday Life", *PLOS ONE*, published online May 11, 2021
Maya Corman, et al., "Attentional Bias Modification With a New Paradigm: The Effect of the Detection Engagement and Savoring Positivity (DESP) Task on Eye-Tracking of Attention", *Journal of Behavior Therapy and Experimental Psychiatry*, 68 (2020): 101525
Kelsey M. Irvin, et al., "The Thrill of Victory: Savoring Positive Affect, Psychophysiological Reward Processing, and Symptoms of Depression", *Emotion*, published online November 30, 2020

Week 35

[1] Yang Bai, et al., "Awe, Daily Stress, and Elevated Life Satisfaction", *Journal of Personality and Social Psychology*, 120 (2021): 837-860
Virginia E. Sturm, et al., "Big Smile, Small Self: Awe Walks Promote Prosocial Positive Emotions in Older Adults", *Emotion*, published online September 21, 2020
Yannick Joye, Jan Willem Bolderdijk, "An Exploratory Study Into the Effects of Extraordinary Nature on Emotions, Mood, and Prosociality", *Frontiers in Psychology*, published online January 28, 2015

Week 36

[1] Katharina Bernecker, Daniela Becker, "Beyond Self-Control: Mechanisms of Hedonic Goal Pursuit and Its Relevance for Well-Being", *Personality and Social Psychology Bulletin*, 47 (2021): 627-642

Week 37

[1] Nicolò F. Bernardi, Antoine Bellemare-Pepin, Isabelle Peretz, "Dancing to 'Groovy' Music Enhances the Experience of Flow", *Annals of the New York Academy of Sciences*, published online May 6, 2018

162

Week 38

[1] Johan G. Ekström, C. Martyn Beaven, "Effects of Blue Light and Caffeine on Mood", *Psychopharmacology*, 231 (2014): 3677-3683

Week 39

[1] Johannes Michalaka, Katharina Rohde, Nikolaus F. Trojec, "How We Walk Affects What We Remember: Gait Modifications Through Biofeedback Change Negative Affective Memory Bias", *Journal of Behavior Therapy and Experimental Psychiatry*, 46 (2015): 121-125

Week 40

[1] Marianna Dalkou, et al., "Can Self-Pampering Act as a Buffer Against Depression in Women? A Cross-Sectional Study", *Health Psychology Research*, 7 (2019): 7967

Week 41

[1] Gregory J. Privitera, Danielle E. Antonelli, Abigail L. Szal, "An Enjoyable Distraction During Exercise Augments the Positive Effects of Exercise on Mood", *Journal of Sports Science & Medicine*, 13 (2014): 266–270

Week 42

[1] Sabine Sonnentag and Cornelia Niessen, "To Detach or Not to Detach? Two Experimental Studies on the Affective Consequences of Detaching From Work During Non-Work Time", *Frontiers in Psychology*, 11 (2020): 560156
Lieke L. ten Brummelhuis, Arnold B. Bakker, "Staying Engaged During the Week: The Effect of Off-Job Activities on Next Day Work Engagement", *Journal of Occupational Health Psychology*, 17 (2012): 445–455
YoungAh Park, Charlotte Fritz, Steve M. Jex, "Relationships Between Work-Home Segmentation and Psychological Detachment From Work: The Role of Communication Technology Use at Home", *Journal of Occupational Health Psychology*, 16 (2011): 457-467
Charlotte Fritz, et al., "Happy, Healthy, and Productive: The Role of Detachment From Work During Non-Work Time", *The Journal of Applied Psychology*, 95 (2010): 977-983

Week 43

[1] Amit Kumar, Matthew A. Killingsworth, Thomas Gilovich, "Spending on Doing Promotes More Moment-to-Moment Happiness Than Spending on Having", *Journal of Experimental Social Psychology*, 88 (2020): 103971

Week 44

[1] Elizabeth B. Raposa, Holly B. Laws, Emily B. Ansell, "Prosocial Behavior Mitigates the Negative Effects of Stress in Everyday Life", *Clinical Psychological Science*, 4 (2016): 691-698
Netta Weinstein, Richard M. Ryan "When Helping Helps: Autonomous Motivation for Prosocial Behavior and Its Influence on Well-Being for the Helper and Recipient", *Journal of Personality and Social Psychology*, 98 (2010): 222-244
Keiko Otake, et al, "Happy People Become Happier Through Kindness: A Counting Kindnesses Intervention", *Journal of Happiness Studies*, 7 (2006): 361-375

[2] Tiantian Mo, et al., "Distressed but Happy: Health Workers and Volunteers During the COVID-19 Pandemic", *Culture and Brain*, Published May 19, 2021

Week 45

[1] Maciej Stolarski, Gerald Matthews, "Time Perspectives Predict Mood States and Satisfaction With Life Over and Above Personality", *Current Psychology*, 35 (2016): 516-526
Jia Wei Zhang, Ryan T. Howell, "Do Time Perspectives Predict Unique Variance in Life Satisfaction Beyond Personality Traits?", *Personality and Individual Differences*, 50 (2011): 1261-1266

Week 46

[1] Tamlin S. Conner, Colin G. DeYoung, Paul J. Silvia, "Everyday Creative Activity as a Path to Flourishing", *The Journal of Positive Psychology*, 13 (2018): 181-189

Week 47

[1] Glenn R. Fox, et al., "Neural Correlates of Gratitude", *Frontiers in Psychology*, 6 (2015): 1491
Roland Zahn, et al., "The Neural Basis of Human Social Values: Evidence From Functional MRI", *Cerebral Cortex*, 19 (2009): 276-283
Michael E. McCullough, Jo-Ann Tsang, Robert A. Emmons, "Gratitude in Intermediate Affective Terrain: Links of Grateful Moods to Individual Differences and Daily Emotional Experience", *Journal of Personality and Social Psychology*, 86 (2004): 295-309

[2] Y. Joel Wong., et al., "Does Gratitude Writing Improve the Mental Health of Psychotherapy Clients? Evidence from a Randomized Controlled Trial", *Psychotherapy Research*, 28 (2018): 192-202

Jane Taylor Wilson, "Brightening the Mind: The Impact of Practicing Gratitude on Focus and Resilience in Learning", *Journal of the Scholarship of Teaching and Learning*, 16 (2016): 1-13

Marta Jackowska, et al., "The Impact of a Brief Gratitude Intervention on Subjective Well-Being, Biology and Sleep", *Journal of Health Psychology*, 21 (2016): 2207-2217

Karen O'Leary, Samantha Dockray, "The Effects of Two Novel Gratitude and Mindfulness Interventions on Well-Being", *Journal of Alternative and Complementary Medicine*, 21 (2015): 243-245

Week 48

[1] Matthias R. Mehl, et al., "Eavesdropping on Happiness: Well-Being Is Related to Having Less Small Talk and More Substantive Conversations", *Psychological Science*, 21 (2010): 539-541

Week 49

[1] Wing-Yee Cheung, et al., "Back to the Future: Nostalgia Increases Optimism", *Personality & Social Psychology Bulletin*, 39 (2013): 1484-1496

Week 50

[1] Marina Iosifyan, Olga Korolkova, "Emotions Associated with Different Textures During Touch", *Consciousness and Cognition*, 71 (2019): 79-85

Week 51

[1] Arif A. Hamid, et al., "Mesolimbic Dopamine Signals the Value of Work", *Nature Neuroscience*, 19 (2016): 117-126

Nico Bunzeck, Emrah Düzel, "Absolute Coding of Stimulus Novelty in the Human Substantia Nigra/VTA", *Neuron*, 51 (2006): 369-379

Week 52

[1] Amanda Lamp, et al., "Exercise, Nutrition, Sleep, and Waking Rest?", *Sleep*, 42 (2019): zsz138

About the Author

Gabrielle Lichterman is a longtime health journalist whose articles have appeared in dozens of major publications around the globe, including *First for Women, Glamour, Marie Claire, New York Daily News, Self, Woman's World* and *Working Mother*. She also served as an editor at **WebMD**.

For more than 20 years, Gabrielle has encouraged her readers to improve their health and well-being by becoming active members of their own healthcare team. By empowering them with important knowledge, trusted studies and unique insight into how to apply this information, she arms readers with the tools they need to create an immediate positive impact in their own lives.

Gabrielle's passion for spreading health empowerment goes beyond the thousands of published articles she's written. Her award-winning book, *28 Days: What Your Cycle Reveals About Your Moods, Health and Potential*, pioneered a new way for women to manage their lives by syncing their activities and health treatments with the hormonal ups and downs in their menstrual cycle. Her popular **Hormonology** method is followed by millions worldwide.

Now Gabrielle is introducing a new technique to help all readers get more from their lives: the **Happiness Upgrade** method. This simple strategy is designed to boost your mood in the moment and can be used virtually anywhere, anytime. Inspired by her own desire to create an on-the-go happiness booster and bolstered by science, the **Happiness Upgrade** method is Gabrielle's latest tool to empower people to improve their own health.

To learn more, visit GabrielleLichterman.com.

CONNECT

 Gabrielle@HappinessUpgradePress.com

 HappinessUpgrade.com

 @happinessupgrade

 @happinessupgrade

 @happinessupgrade

 @happinessupgrad

Made in the USA
Columbia, SC
13 April 2022

58665190R00098